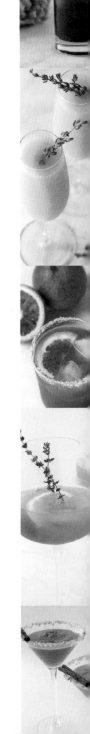

MOCKTAIL PARTY

75 Plant-Based, Non-Alcoholic Mocktail Recipes for Every Occasion

Kerry Benson, MS, RD, LDN, and Diana Licalzi, MS, RD, CDCES

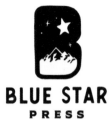

BLUE STAR
P R E S S

Photography by Kerry Benson and Diana Licalzi Maldonado
Cover and Interior Design by Rhoda Wong

ISBN 9781950968244

Printed in Colombia

10 9 8 7 6

DISCLAIMER:
This book is for informational and educational purposes. This book is not intended to be a substitute for the medical advice of a licensed physician. The reader should consult with their doctor in any matters relating to their health.

The information in this book is not intended to treat, diagnose, cure, or prevent disease. This book is not sponsored or endorsed by any organization or company. The information in this book is based on experience and research done by the authors. Neither the publisher nor the authors accept any liability of any kind for any damages caused, directly or indirectly, from the use of the information in this book.

DEDICATION

This book would not have been possible without the
love and support of our significant others, families,
and friends. We are grateful for your encouragement
and your discerning taste buds.

CONTENTS

1 — CLASSICS

2 — WITH A TWIST

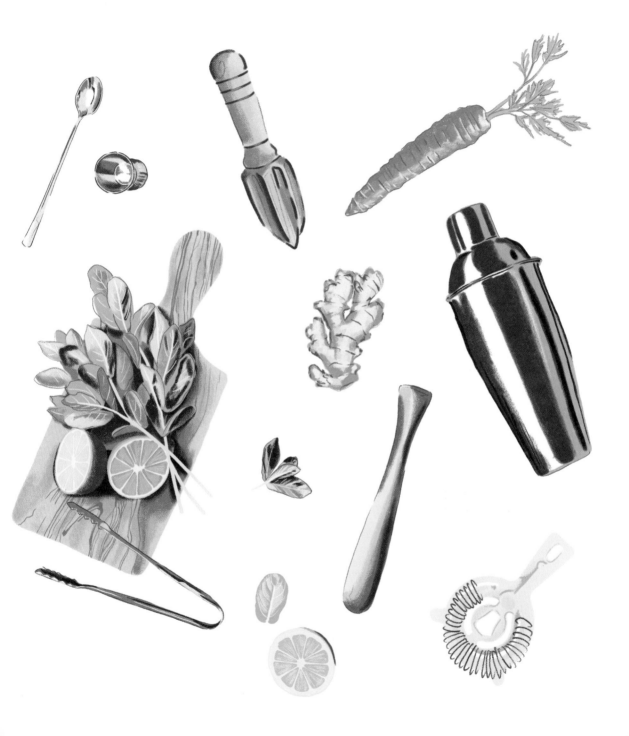

INTRODUCTION

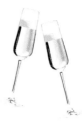

We are a culture that loves to drink.

We toast special moments and holidays with alcohol, but we also drink because it's brunch, because we've had a hard day at work, or because we're binge-watching reality TV. Alcohol is ubiquitous. This is changing, though, thanks to the "sober curious" movement and challenges such as Dry January and Sober October.

If you picked up this book, you're probably interested in cutting back on or eliminating alcohol, either temporarily or permanently. Some people are looking to reset after overindulging during the holidays, while others are trying to get pregnant or make a lifestyle change. But if you give up the sauce, how do you fill the void? Seltzer water is great, especially with all the fun flavors out there these days. But is that enough to make you feel included at a party, or to quench your thirst for a glass of crisp rosé wine on a hot summer evening? Probably not!

That's where we come in. We are Kerry and Diana, registered dietitians and the authors of *Drinking for Two: Nutritious Mocktails for the Mom-to-Be*. After publishing our first book, we noticed a growing demand for a version that would appeal to all audiences, not just expecting mothers. So, we got back into the kitchen and created this collection of original, plant-based mocktail recipes perfect for anyone looking to cut back on booze.

What makes *Mocktail Party* unique compared to other mocktail books on the shelves? Written by two credentialed health professionals, this book offers drinks that are both delicious and nutritious. Mocktails and their alcoholic counterparts can be very juice-heavy and are often loaded with sugar, syrup, and other undesirable ingredients. We keep added sugar to a minimum and instead rely on all-natural ingredients like coconut water, herbs, spices, teas, and whole fruits to add flavor and sweetness.

All of our drinks are plant-based, but they can easily be adapted to accommodate any dietary preferences or restrictions. They also include everyday ingredients that you can find at your local food store, and most can be whipped up in just a matter of minutes! We extensively tested all the beverages in this book, so you can feel confident that each recipe will yield a tasty mocktail.

From a quiet dinner at home to a summer barbeque to a holiday party, our mocktails are the perfect addition to any occasion. Let's get this party started. Cheers!

WHY MOVE TO MOCKTAILS?

When we think about health and nutrition, we often focus on what we eat rather than what we put in our glasses. But what we drink is just as important! In this chapter, we review the complex relationship between alcohol and health. We also highlight two common components of mocktails—added sugar and juice—and explain how we mindfully use these ingredients in this book.

ALCOHOL AND HEALTH

From a nutrition perspective, ethanol, commonly referred to as alcohol, contributes seven calories per gram without any nutrient value; in other words, alcohol provides "empty calories." A standard drink that has about 14 grams of alcohol will set you back roughly 100 calories, not including any additional calories from other components like the carbohydrates in beer or the simple syrup in a cocktail. Thus, alcohol consumption can lead to increased calorie intake and, in turn, weight gain. Excess alcohol intake negatively impacts digestion and nutrient absorption, and in extreme cases, can lead to nutrient deficiencies. For example, chronic alcohol abuse can deplete B vitamins, namely thiamin (B1), which may cause permanent neurological damage.

TERMINOLOGY

Moderate drinking: 2 drinks per day for men, 1 drink per day for women
Heavy drinking: 15 or more drinks per week for men, 8 or more drinks per week for women
Binge drinking: 5 or more drinks on one occasion for men, 4 or more drinks on one occasion for women
Excessive drinking: includes heavy drinking, binge drinking, and any alcohol consumption by pregnant women or individuals under the age of 21

The terms below describing patterns of drinking were obtained from the CDC and NIAAA websites. Organizations and research studies may not use consistent definitions.

1 standard drink = 14 grams alcohol
5 fluid ounces (1 glass) wine, 12% ABV
12 fluid ounces (1 can or bottle) beer, 5% ABV
1½ fluid ounces (1 shot) liquor, 40% ABV

Most of us are aware that excessive alcohol consumption may result in negative health outcomes, both in the short and long term (see Appendix 1 for more information). But what about moderate alcohol consumption?

The American Heart Association, American Cancer Society, and 2020–2025 Dietary Guidelines for Americans all state that individuals who choose to drink should limit their intake to no more than two standard drinks per day for men and one drink per day for women. The scientific report released by the Dietary Guidelines Advisory Comittee stated that "drinking less is better for health than drinking more" and proposed "tightening" the limits for alcohol consumption to one drink per day for both men and women. The National Institute on Alcohol Abuse and Alcoholism (NIAAA) recommends men over the age of 65 limit alcohol intake to one drink per day as well. And no, this does not mean you can save all your drinks for the weekend!

Some literature suggests that moderate alcohol consumption may be beneficial to health. For example, studies have demonstrated that moderate drinking is associated with a decreased risk of type 2 diabetes and cardiovascular disease. Many of us have also heard about the potential heart-healthy benefits of red wine, and a body of evidence supports this claim. For example, one to two glasses of red wine per day has been associated with benefits such as increased HDL, or "good cholesterol." Red wine also contains resveratrol and other antioxidants, which may improve various markers of cardiovascular health.

On the other hand, some evidence suggests a negative relationship between light to moderate alcohol consumption and health. For example, any amount of alcohol consumption increases the risk of certain types of cancer, such as esophageal cancer. Moderate alcohol intake has also been associated with an increased risk of breast cancer. A recent study examined data from nearly 600,000 individuals from nineteen high-income countries and found that, among current drinkers, consuming more than five to six "standard" drinks per week was associated with an increased risk of mortality.

Like many topics in nutrition research, it is challenging to study the relationship between alcohol and health. Many studies are observational, meaning that individuals are followed over time. In this type of study design, a relationship between two variables may be found, but it can be difficult to know the cause and effect. For example, does moderate alcohol intake decrease the risk of chronic disease, or do people who have a lower risk of chronic disease tend to drink more moderately? In addition, other variables like demographics, genetics, and lifestyle factors may influence observed associations between alcohol intake and health. For example, do people who drink red wine eat differently than those who don't, and to what extent does this explain the relationship between red wine intake and health? Overall, it is hard to draw firm conclusions from the existing data.

Are you ready for some good news? Taking even a short break from alcohol may provide many health benefits. For example, an observational study in London found that abstinence from alcohol for one month in moderate-heavy drinkers was associated with improved insulin resistance, lower blood pressure, and weight loss. While other lifestyle changes, like diet, may have contributed to these outcomes, the results are nevertheless compelling. What's more, many of the participants who abstained from drinking for a month stayed the course, eliminating or reducing alcohol for an additional six to eight months after the end of the study. There was also a significant reduction in the percent of individuals engaging in "harmful" drinking behaviors.

Always consult with your healthcare provider for individualized guidance on alcohol consumption. Some individuals should refrain from drinking alcohol completely, including those who are underage, individuals taking certain medications or managing medical conditions, those in recovery, and women who are pregnant or trying to conceive. The topic of drinking during pregnancy is very close to our hearts, which is why we developed a mocktail recipe book aimed at expectant mothers called *Drinking for Two: Nutritious Mocktails for the Mom-to-Be*.

Overall, most of us could benefit from swapping at least some of our cocktails for mocktails. We think this "sober curious" trend is here to stay, and we are all about it! We're here to provide you with recipes that look and taste the part while using easy-to-find, nutritious ingredients and keeping added sugars to a minimum.

Note: Even though our mocktails are a healthier alternative to cocktails, you should still follow the guidance of your healthcare provider or sponsor before you make mocktails a part of your regular routine.

ADDED SUGARS

Added sugars are not naturally found in foods; instead, they are added during processing. Check the ingredient list, and you may find added sugar under the guise of dextrose, brown rice syrup, high fructose corn syrup, and many other names. Natural sweeteners like honey, agave nectar, maple syrup, coconut sugar, and molasses are still considered sources of added sugar even though they are less processed and may have some nutritional value.

Added sugars easily sneak into our diets, especially our drinks. Cocktails and mocktails often contain different forms of sugar, including simple syrup, soda or tonic water, ginger beer, or conventional white sugar. We've seen some mocktail recipes that contain as much as 1 ounce of sweetener in a single drink serving. That's 2 tablespoons, or 6 teaspoons, of sugar per serving—and that's not including sugars from other ingredients, such as juice or soda!

One ounce may not sound like a lot, but how does this compare to the guidelines on added sugar intake? The 2020–2025 Dietary Guidelines for Americans recommends limiting added sugar to less than 10% of calories. For someone consuming 2,000 calories a day, this is less than 50 grams per day, or 12 teaspoons (1 teaspoon = 4 grams sugar = 16 calories). The American Heart Association (AHA) recommendations are more stringent: Added sugar consumption should be limited to 6 teaspoons a day for women and 9 teaspoons for men. Using the example above, just one drink could put you at or close to the maximum recommended intake of added sugar for the day!

Minimizing added sugars is important for several reasons. Like alcohol, they are a source of "empty calories" that provide little to no nutritional value. Added sugar either displaces more nutrient-dense sources of calories or contributes to an increase in overall calorie intake, which can lead to overeating and weight gain. In addition, both added sugars and refined grains elevate blood sugar levels more than fruits, vegetables, and whole grains, which contain fiber. Fiber slows digestion and absorption of nutrients, namely glucose, into the bloodstream. Thus, fiber-containing foods are less likely to cause a spike in blood sugar.

We limit added sugar in our recipes, and when we do include it, we opt for natural sweeteners. We use ingredients like herbs, spices, and fruit to add flavor and sweetness to the greatest extent possible.

SUGAR SUBSTITUTES

Sugar substitutes, or non-nutritive sweeteners (NNS), are commonly used to add a sweet taste to food or drinks with few to no calories. NNS can be categorized into two groups—artificial and natural. Artificial sweeteners and their brand names include aspartame (Equal), saccharin (Sweet'N Low), and sucralose (Splenda)—and as their name implies, these sweeteners are artificially made through chemical processes. Natural NNS and their brand names include stevia leaf extract (e.g. Stevia in the Raw) and monk fruit extract (e.g., Lakanto).

These sweeteners may be sugar-free, but this doesn't mean that they are "healthy." NNS are up to 150 to 700 times sweeter than regular sugar. Frequent use of these sweeteners can overstimulate your taste receptors, meaning you may find naturally sweet foods like fruit less appealing and, therefore, may need more sweetness to satisfy you. What's more, recent research seems to suggest that NNS may negatively impact the gut microbiome. On the other hand, smart use of NNS can help reduce the intake of added sugar, contributing to healthy body weight. This, in turn, may reduce the risk of chronic diseases, such as diabetes and heart disease. Overall, the consensus seems to be that occasionally enjoying these sweeteners is perfectly OK.

We prefer natural NNS to artificial, and we tested a few of our recipes with monk fruit sweetener. We found that monk fruit sweetener tastes delicious in our drinks and doesn't leave you with an unpleasant aftertaste like stevia sometimes does. If it aligns better with your health goals, feel free to use non-nutritive sweeteners in place of agave nectar, honey, etc. in our drinks!

TO JUICE OR NOT TO JUICE?

Most Americans do not eat enough fruits and vegetables, and may rely on 100% juices to help meet micronutrient needs. to meet their micronutrient needs. Fruit juice is convenient, inexpensive, and contains antioxidants and other non-nutritive plant components, such as polyphenols, that may be beneficial for health. However, juice consumption is controversial because it is high in natural sugar without the benefit of the fiber naturally present in whole fruits.

Health professionals are divided on whether drinking juice is "healthy." As with many areas in nutrition, more research is needed (surprise, surprise). Note that juice cocktails, nectars, and other juices with added sugars do not fall under this umbrella and should be avoided.

We chose to include freshly squeezed and 100% juices in our recipes because we believe they serve a purpose, not the least of which is adding flavor and color to drinks. Most of our drink recipes include no more than a few ounces of juice, if any, and many are made with whole fruits.

Like cocktails, our drinks should be consumed in moderation but can have a place in a healthy lifestyle. When developing our recipes, we took measures to minimize or completely avoid adding sugar, syrup, and alternative sweeteners. And don't forget that you're saving quite a few calories just by eliminating alcohol!

TOOLS AND TECHNIQUES

Now, let's get your kitchen set up so that you can make a mocktail whenever the mood strikes! In this chapter, we review the kitchen appliances, tools, and glassware you'll need and teach you a few basic bartending techniques.

If making a mocktail seems intimidating, don't fret. Our drink recipes are easier to prepare than you might think—no prior bartending experience required. Most of the mocktails in this book only take a few minutes to throw together and use ingredients and methods that are probably familiar to you.

Proper tools are essential to make any recipe, and mocktails are no exception. The good news is that you may have most of these tools and appliances in your kitchen already. If not, and you prefer not to buy anything, we provide suggestions and alternatives when we can.

HIGH-POWERED BLENDER
A high-powered blender is necessary to prepare many of our mocktails, namely those that are frozen. For smaller quantities or softer ingredients, a food processor works fine, too.

SHAKER
A shaker helps to mix and cool ingredients with the addition of ice. It also serves as a great holder for muddling. There are two types of shakers: the cobbler shaker and the Boston shaker. A cobbler shaker, commonly referred to as a 3-piece cocktail shaker, has a built-in strainer and is often used by beginners. A Boston shaker comes with two cups—either two metal tumblers or one metal tumbler and one tempered glass—as well as a separate strainer, either a Hawthorne or julep strainer. Bartenders often favor the Boston shaker because it holds more liquid, making it more efficient when dealing with a busy crowd. Either one works for making a mocktail. If you don't want to purchase a shaker, feel free to improvise. Find a shaker lid for Mason or Ball jars, use a travel coffee mug, or as a last resort, reach for a reusable water bottle—we used all of these at some point while creating these recipes!

FINE-MESH STRAINER, CHEESECLOTH, OR NUT MILK BAG
We like to offer you the option of "pulp or no pulp" in a few of our drinks. A fine-mesh strainer, cheesecloth, or nut milk bag can be used interchangeably to strain out any unde-sired ingredient bits. In many cases, straining helps to create a picture-perfect mocktail, but if you include the pulp, you will get a nutritional boost in the form of fiber.

MUDDLER

Muddling is a technique we frequently use throughout the book, as it helps bring out the flavor of fresh fruit and herbs. A muddler is a long bar tool with an enlarged tip, usually made of wood or steel. Either type of muddler works for our recipes. You can find muddlers online or buy one wherever you normally find basic kitchen tools. If buying a muddler is not an option, you can use the back of a mixing spoon instead.

CITRUS JUICER

A citrus juicer can be handy for preparing freshly squeezed citrus juice, such as lemon or lime. You can order a basic citrus juicer online for less than ten dollars, or pick one up anywhere basic kitchen tools are sold. Prefer not to buy a citrus juicer? Put those hands to work and squeeze. Or, stick with bottled juice—just look for one with no added sugar or preservatives.

REUSABLE OR RECYCLABLE STRAWS

Not a must-have, but straws are a fun addition to mocktails and can make some drinks, like our frozen ones, easier to sip. To be environmentally friendly, we suggest purchasing bamboo, paper, or metal straws.

GLASSWARE

Using appropriate glassware enhances the experience of drinking a mocktail. In our recipes, we note which type of glass is best suited for that particular drink. Here is a list of the glassware that we use throughout the book:

Highball glasses (e.g., for our Mock-jitos)
Lowball glasses (e.g., for our Mock-a-ritas)
   • Stemless wine glasses serve as a good substitute.
Champagne glasses (for sparkling drinks)
Wine glasses (e.g., for our Sans-gria drinks)
Martini or coupe glasses (e.g., for our Mock-tinis)
Copper mugs (for Mocktail Mules)
   • Don't have these on hand? Substitute with lowball or stemless wine glasses.
Hurricane or other large glasses (for tropical, frozen drinks)
Standard mugs (for warm beverages)
Pitcher or large vessel for mixing or serving

The quantities of our drinks are designed to fit standard glassware. If you find that one serving of the drink does not quite fill your glass, you may be using a glass that is larger than the standard size. We felt that it was important to stick with "standard" drink quantities to give you a similar experience to having an alcoholic drink and to keep portions in check.

You may note differences in the number of servings each recipe yields throughout the book. We chose the number of servings for each drink based on the preparation method, ingredients required, and occasion. For example, our shaken mocktails make two servings, while many of our frozen, blended drink recipes prepare four or more servings. Feel free to adjust the quantity based on the availability of ingredients and the size of your shaker, blender, or other equipment.

MEASURING CUPS AND SPOONS

Drink recipes are typically written in ounces. However, to simplify matters, we decided to use more common units of measure, like teaspoons and cups. Hence, you may come across quantities like "2 tablespoons and 2 teaspoons" instead of "1.3 ounces."

HOW-TOs

We're nutrition professionals, not mixologists, and had no bartending experience prior to writing our mocktail books. Here are some basic techniques we learned along the way—and if we can learn them, trust us, so can you!

HOW TO USE A SHAKER

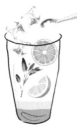 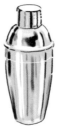 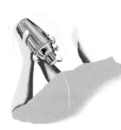 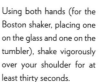 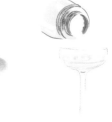

Pour your ingredients into the shaker (or glass if using the Boston shaker) and add ice, unless indicated otherwise. Note: some recipes call for "dry shaking," which means shaking ingredients without the addition of ice.

Depending on what shaker you are using, place the lid or metal tumbler on securely. The one pictured above is a cobbler shaker.

For the Boston shaker, make sure that the top metal tumbler is well sealed to the bottom glass by tapping the bottom of the tumbler with the heel of your hand.

Using both hands (for the Boston shaker, placing one on the glass and one on the tumbler), shake vigorously over your shoulder for at least thirty seconds.

Strain the mixture into glasses.

For the cobbler shaker, you will be able to strain through the top piece of the shaker. For the Boston shaker, you will use a separate strainer. To break the seal between the top and bottom glasses before straining, use the heel of your hand to tap the rim of the glass carefully but assertively. This may take a few tries.

HOW TO MUDDLE

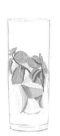

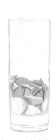

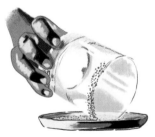

Place herbs and/or fruit at the bottom of a glass or shaker.

Using a muddler, gently press down on the herbs and/or fruit and twist three or four times.

The goal is to slightly bruise the herbs but not break them; a good way to measure this is through smell. For example, if your mint starts to smell minty, you're in great shape!

HOW TO RIM A GLASS

Rims are often an essential part of the experience of drinking a mocktail. Rimming a glass is a great way to enhance flavors—hello, salted Margaritas!

Dry ingredients are the ingredients placed on the rim. In this book, you'll see salt for Margaritas and crushed nuts or graham crackers for various dessert drinks. Use a plate or shallow bowl to hold your dry ingredients.

Wet ingredients are used to stick the dry ingredients to the rim. We use several methods to wet the rim of a glass. These include sliding a lime wedge or piece of fruit around the rim, or pouring a liquid like maple syrup in a plate or shallow bowl and then dipping the rim. You can also use your fingers to apply the wet ingredient to the glass.

After wetting the rim, dip and twist! Turn the glass upside down and dip its moistened rim into your dry mixture. Gently twist the glass. Repeat until the rim is covered with the desired amount of dry ingredients.

ESSENTIAL INGREDIENTS

In this section, we provide you with a list of basic ingredients to have on hand, so when the urge to make a mocktail hits, you'll be ready! We avoided creating recipes with obscure, hard-to-find ingredients. Bonus: many of the ingredients can be used for multiple recipes.

The good news is that our recipes are easily adaptable, so feel free to get creative and try other ingredients. With that said, we can't guarantee the same results (taste, look, etc.) if you depart from the written recipes. We spent a lot of time testing and trying different ingredients, methods, and quantities, and what we provide in this book is the fruit of our efforts. Also, if you're like us and hate wasting leftover ingredients, don't worry! We offer tips and ideas for how to use extra ingredients throughout the book, as well as in Appendix 4.

SELTZER WATER
There are three basic types of carbonated water: sparkling mineral water, seltzer, and club soda. We recommend seltzer for our recipes as it's typically cheaper than its alternatives and is strongly carbonated. We use plain seltzer, with no added flavors or sweeteners. As you have probably experienced, any type of carbonated water will become flat when it is left open for an extended period, so always use fresh carbonated water for drinks.

COCONUT WATER
Coconut water is used in many of our recipes. Coconut water contains electrolytes, such as potassium, and has a natural sweetness. Avoid brands that add additional sugar by checking to make sure it's not listed in the ingredients. For some drinks, we provide the alternative option of using maple water. Similar to coconut water, maple water is naturally sweet and contains electrolytes, but it has a different flavor that we felt would lend itself to certain recipes. Maple water can be difficult to find, but coconut water works well as a substitute.

JUICE
Many of our recipes contain juice, from citrus to pomegranate to grape. We recommend freshly squeezed juice over bottled, as it's more flavorful and free of preservatives. However, when preparing mocktails in larger quantities, purchasing bottled juice is perfectly fine. Opt for 100% juice with no added sugar and choose juice in glass bottles. When squeezing fresh juice, wash and dry the fruits well before cutting into them, and use immediately.

In our recipes, we use readily available cranberry juice, as it's 100% juice made with grape and/or apple juice for sweetness; 100% cranberry juice is not the same and is extremely tart. Avoid "cranberry juice cocktails."

Throughout the book, we tell you how many tablespoons or cups of citrus juice to add to a drink. Below, we provide a reference for how much fruit you need to squeeze to get that amount of juice. This will vary with the size and ripeness of your fruit, but hopefully it will give you a sense of how much fruit to have on hand.

Lemon
1 lemon = 2 tablespoons juice

Lime
1 lime = 2 tablespoons juice

Orange
1 orange = 1/4 cup juice

Grapefruit
1 grapefruit = 1/2 cup juice

GINGER

Ginger adds a spicy, zesty flavor to many of our mocktails. Some of our recipes may say "1 teaspoon peeled and chopped ginger." This simply means peel the outer skin off the ginger using a peeler, paring knife, or spoon, chop it into pieces, and then measure in a teaspoon. Depending on how well your blender works, the ginger may or may not blend into small, unnoticeable pieces. You can always strain out any large pieces or, better yet, leave them in your drink for a nutritional boost! Ginger can stay fresh for about a week at room temperature and close to a month in the refrigerator. Please note, ground ginger has a much more concentrated flavor than fresh ginger and will not work well as a replacement in our recipes.

FRESH HERBS

Fresh herbs, such as mint, basil, and thyme, are used in many of our recipes. Herbs offer a range of nutritional benefits and add wonderful flavor to drinks. Unfortunately, herbs tend to go bad rather quickly, so it's best to buy them when you plan to make a mocktail—or better yet, try growing your own herbs at home! You may have bought herbs before and had to toss a decent amount away. To avoid this, look for the fun tips and recipe ideas for using leftover herbs found in the main chapters and Appendix 4.

NON-DAIRY MILK

You'll see "non-dairy milk" in a handful of our recipes. Feel free to use your favorite: almond, oat, coconut, soy, or any other non-dairy milk. Most non-dairy milks can be used interchangeably in these recipes unless stated otherwise (e.g., we recommend coconut milk for the Piña Col-nada). We recommend buying unsweetened, unflavored non-dairy milks (as opposed to those flavored with vanilla) and adding vanilla extract when it is called for, as this will create a stronger, tastier flavor.

COCONUT MILK

Coconut milk comes in different package types (can or carton) and different concentrations (regular or light). Canned is richer than carton, and, of course, regular is richer than light; added water makes the difference.

We use canned coconut milk in small quantities to add richness and a creamy texture to some of our drinks. We chose the regular kind as opposed to the light version for taste and texture purposes. You'll often find canned coconut milk in the ethnic foods section of your grocery store. When canned coconut milk sits out for a while, the contents may separate. We recommend either giving it a good shake or blending it up in a food processor before using.

Coconut milk in a carton is generally found alongside other non-dairy beverages and is watered down to the greatest extent. In our recipes, we always specify which type of coconut milk to use, canned or carton, to help you avoid confusion.

FRESH OR FROZEN FRUIT

We developed drink recipes that incorporate whole fruits whenever possible to preserve the fruit's nutritional content, namely fiber. You'll see a range of fruits, including berries, bananas, and pineapples in our recipes. We often give you the option to use fresh or frozen fruit. Frozen fruit has the same nutritional value as fresh fruit, and you don't have to worry about it going bad. Keep frozen blueberries, strawberries, mango, and pineapple on hand. You can even peel, slice up, and freeze ripe bananas for later use. Always wash fresh produce well before consuming.

DATES

You may notice dates in a few of our recipes. Dates are a naturally sweet fruit packed with lots of nutrients. Dates provide antioxidants, fiber, and micronutrients, like potassium and vitamin B6. When there's an opportunity to blend a drink, we choose dates as our sweetener so you can reap the benefits of their nutritional content while enjoying their sweetness. We prefer Medjool dates, but other dates will work fine. Soaking the dates in water for about 10 minutes prior to blending helps to soften them up and facilitates blending.

SWEETENERS

For a handful of recipes, we needed to add a touch of sweetness but couldn't use dates for various reasons. For example, the drink didn't require blending, or we found that the dates changed the flavor or color too much. Instead, we used a small amount of agave nectar, honey, or maple syrup. We keep the quantities to a minimum, but feel free to adjust the sweetness according to your preference. Agave nectar, honey, and maple syrup can be used interchangeably, but we do specify which sweetener we used when testing our drinks to best complement certain flavors. As discussed in Why Move to Mocktails, you can substitute monk fruit sweetener for the added sugar in our recipes for a reduced-calorie variation.

APPLE CIDER VINEGAR

Yes, we use apple cider vinegar in our drinks! We found it adds a "bite" similar to that of alcohol, and helps to balance the sweetness from juice. We use minimal amounts, so don't worry about it being overpowering.

VANILLA AND OTHER EXTRACTS

Vanilla and other commonly used extracts are typically prepared in alcohol. For a product to be considered vanilla "extract," the FDA requires an alcohol content of at least 35% by volume (in 1 teaspoon of extract, there may be 1/3 teaspoon of alcohol, or 0.056 ounces). These extracts are commonly used in baking, and the alcohol evaporates when it is heated.

We use these extracts in small quantities (no more than 1 teaspoon per serving) in our drinks to add flavor. If you want to avoid alcohol completely, we suggest substituting a non-alcoholic version. Better yet, use real vanilla bean (1 teaspoon extract = one 2-inch piece of vanilla bean) or vanilla bean paste, though vanilla beans are expensive. You can also use flavored, unsweetened non-dairy milk to add vanilla flavor to some drinks, such as our mock-tinis.

CHAPTER

1

CLASSICS

Let's get down to basics. In this section, we give you mocktail versions of some of your favorite classic cocktails, like the Margarita, Aperol Spritz, and Cosmopolitan—all with a reduced-sugar makeover.

APEROL-LESS SPRITZ

SERVES 4

While the colors may not resemble a typical Aperol Spritz, our mocktail version still captures the signature sweet and bitter flavors. Citrusy and herbaceous, our Aperol-less Spritz is well-balanced and perfect for a summer evening!

INGREDIENTS

2 sprigs fresh thyme

4 sage leaves

2 teaspoons lemon juice

1 cup orange juice

½ cup grapefruit juice

½ cup pomegranate juice

½ cup white grape juice

1 teaspoon apple cider vinegar

2 cups seltzer

Extra herbs and orange slices or peel for garnish

TOOLS

Muddler

Pitcher

PREPARATION

1. Gently muddle the fresh thyme and sage with the lemon juice in the bottom of a pitcher.

2. Add all the remaining ingredients except the seltzer to the pitcher. Stir. This can be done ahead of time!

3. Fill four wine glasses with ice and divide the mixture among the glasses. Top with seltzer (½ cup per serving).

4. Garnish with extra herbs and add a twist of orange peel or orange slices to each glass.

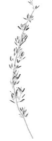

USE EXTRA HERBS TO ADD FLAVOR TO ROASTED FRESH VEGETABLES. SAGE AND THYME PAIR WELL TOGETHER IN MANY DISHES!

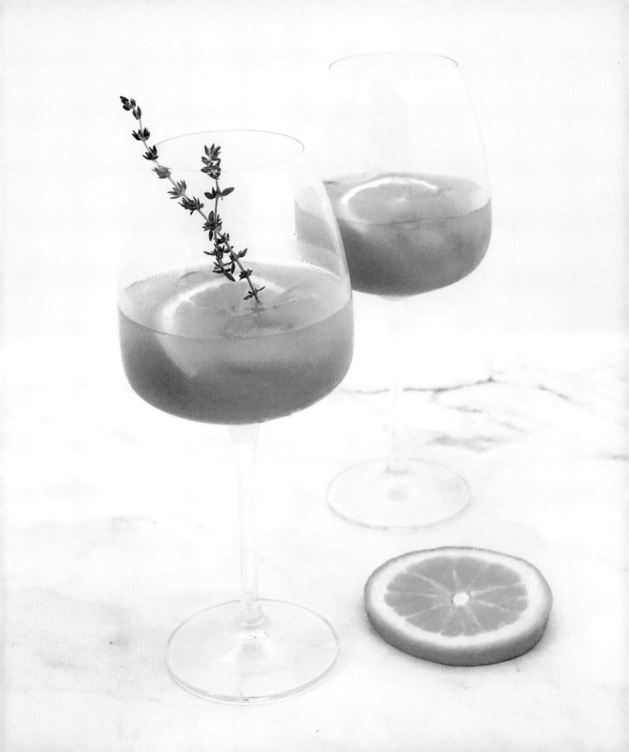

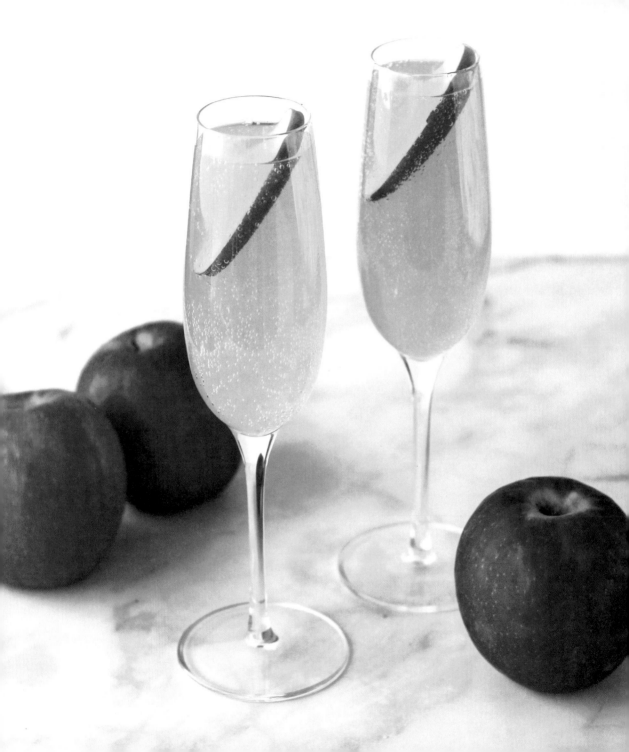

SPARKLING CIDER

If you're craving a crisp, cool cider without the alcohol, this drink will certainly do the trick. Change up your glassware to fit the occasion. Use a highball glass if you are feeling like a casual cider drink, or serve in a champagne glass to toast a special moment!

INGREDIENTS

2 cups 100% apple juice

¼ cup orange juice

2 teaspoons apple cider vinegar

2 ⅔ cups seltzer

TOOLS

Pitcher

PREPARATION

1. Combine all the ingredients except the seltzer in a pitcher. Stir.

2. Divide the mixture among four highball or champagne glasses.

3. Top with seltzer (⅔ cup per serving).

FOR A FALL VERSION, MUDDLE SOME FRESH GINGER IN THE BOTTOM OF THE PITCHER BEFORE ADDING THE REMAINING INGREDIENTS, AND ADD A COUPLE OF SHAKES OF GROUND CINNAMON AND NUTMEG.

PAL-NO-MA

A Paloma is a tequila-based cocktail made with grapefruit soda. Our mocktail gets its natural sweetness from coconut water and a hint of honey or agave nectar, and its tartness from grapefruit juice.

INGREDIENTS

SALTED RIM

Lime wedges

Sea salt

DRINK

1 cup coconut or maple water

½ cup grapefruit juice

¼ cup lime juice

2 teaspoons apple cider vinegar

2 teaspoons honey or agave nectar

Dash of salt

½ cup seltzer

Grapefruit or lime slices for garnish

TOOLS

Shaker

PREPARATION

1. Rim two lowball or margarita glasses with salt (see page 10).

2. Combine all the ingredients except the seltzer in a shaker, and add ice. Shake vigorously for 30 seconds.

3. Strain the shaken mixture into the two rimmed glasses.

4. Top with seltzer (1/4 cup per serving). Stir.

5. Garnish with grapefruit or lime slices.

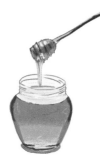

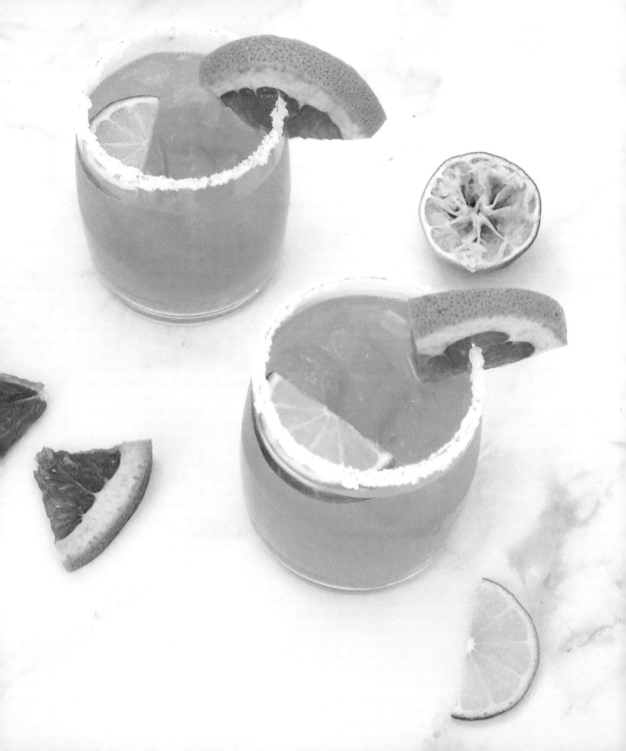

BASIC MOCK-JITO

Our take on the classic Cuban cocktail gets natural sweetness from coconut water and an "alcoholic" bite from the apple cider vinegar. Refreshing and perfect on a hot day!

INGREDIENTS

20 mint leaves

2 lime wedges

2 teaspoons agave nectar

1 teaspoon apple cider vinegar

⅔ cup coconut water

1 cup seltzer

Additional mint sprigs or leaves for garnish

TOOLS

Muddler

Shaker

PREPARATION

1. Muddle the mint leaves and lime wedges with the agave nectar and apple cider vinegar in the bottom of a shaker.

2. Add coconut water and ice. Shake vigorously.

3. Divide the shaken mixture, including the muddled mint, lime wedges, and ice, evenly between the glasses. Top with additional ice as desired.

4. Top with seltzer (½ cup per serving) and stir.

5. Garnish with mint sprigs.

USE EXTRA MINT TO BREW MINT TEA, OR USE IT IN A WATERMELON, FETA, AND MINT SALAD!

ZERO-PROOF SPARKLING WINE

SERVES 4

Toast special occasions with this non-alcoholic sparkling wine, made with antioxidant-rich and easy-to-find ingredients.

INGREDIENTS

1 cup white grape juice or pomegranate juice

½ cup coconut or maple water

2 tablespoons and 2 teaspoons lemon juice

1 tablespoon and 1 teaspoon apple cider vinegar

2 cups seltzer

TOOLS

Pitcher

PREPARATION

1. Combine all the ingredients except the seltzer in a pitcher. Stir.

2. Divide the mixture among four wine or champagne glasses.

3. Top with seltzer (½ cup per serving).

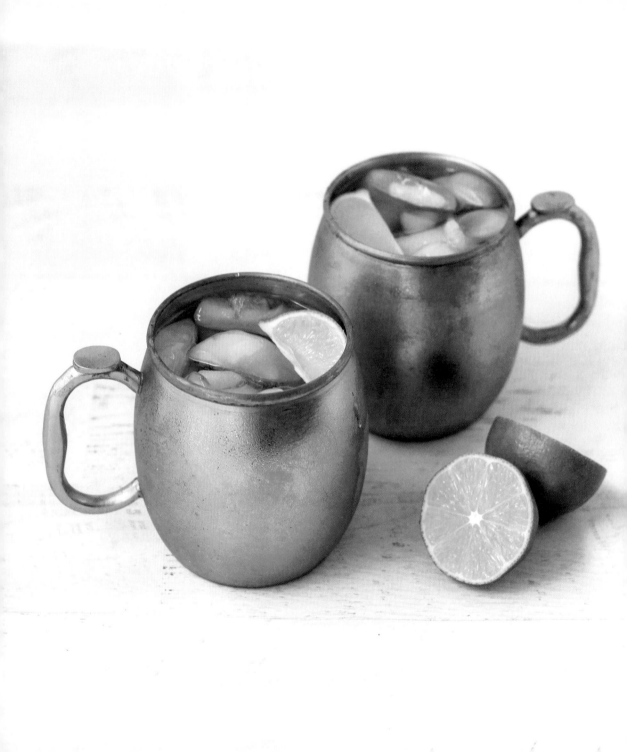

MOCKTAIL MULE

In this mocktail, ginger-flavored kombucha serves as a nutritious and functional swap for ginger beer—one of the main components of a Moscow Mule.

INGREDIENTS

2 ⅔ cups ginger-flavored kombucha

¼ cup lime juice

2 cups seltzer

Lime wedges for garnish

TOOLS

Pitcher

PREPARATION

1. Combine all the ingredients in a pitcher. Stir.

2. Fill four copper mugs with ice and divide the mixture between the glasses.

3. Garnish with lime wedges.

PREGNANT WOMEN SHOULD CONSUME KOMBUCHA WITH CAUTION. SEE APPENDIX 2.

SOUR MOCK-A-RITA

SERVES 4-6

What could be better than a classic Margarita? How about a hangover-proof version? Our Sour Mock-a-rita has all the flavor of the original beverage plus hydrating coconut water, with minimal added sugar.

INGREDIENTS

SALTED RIM

Lime wedges

Sea salt

DRINK

1 cup and 2 tablespoons lime juice

¼ cup and 2 tablespoons orange juice

3 tablespoons agave nectar, plus more to taste

2½ cups and 2 tablespoons coconut water

Few dashes of salt

Lime wheels for garnish

TOOLS

Pitcher

PREPARATION

1. Salt the rims of four to six lowball or margarita glasses (see page 10).

2. Combine all the drink ingredients in a pitcher. Stir.

3. Fill the rimmed glasses with ice and divide the mixture among the glasses.

4. Garnish with lime wheels.

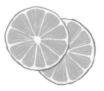

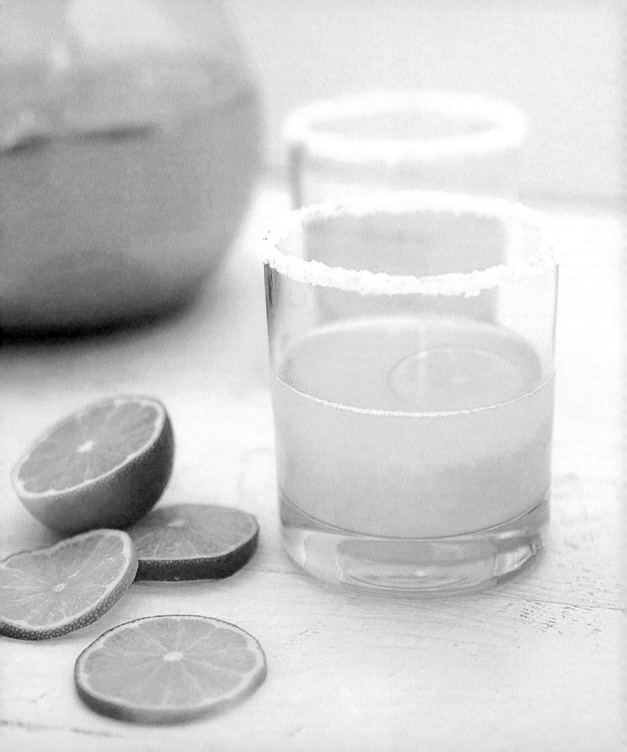

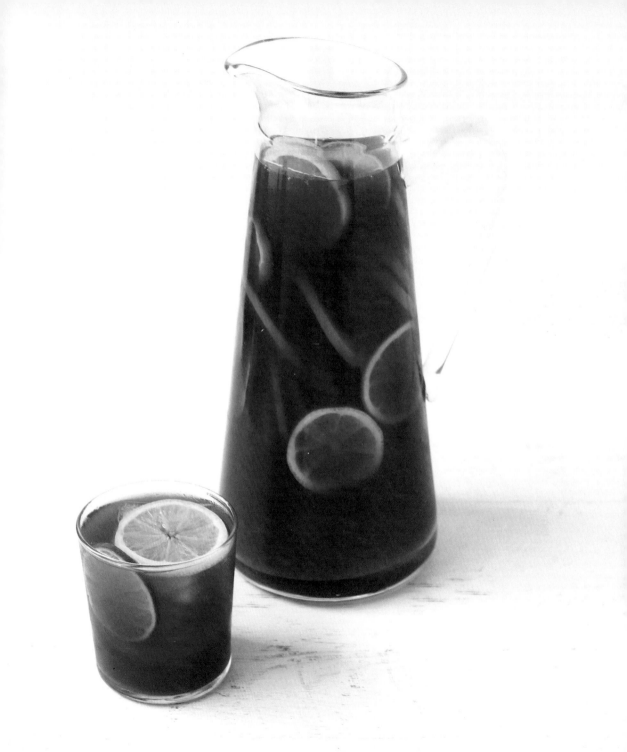

RED SANS-GRIA

Perfect for large groups, our Red Sans-gria is one of our most popular recipes. Feel free to use whatever fruit you like based on the occasion or season. Add fresh herbs or spices for another layer of flavor!

INGREDIENTS

1 lemon with peel, thinly sliced

1 lime with peel, thinly sliced

1 medium orange with peel, thinly sliced

1 small apple with peel, cored and sliced into eighths

2 ½ cups 100% pomegranate juice (no sugar added) or grape juice (or a combination of the two!)

2 ½ cups coconut water

1 cup orange juice

¼ cup lime juice

TOOLS

Muddler

Pitcher

PREPARATION

1. Combine all the sliced fruit in a large pitcher. Muddle.

2. Add the pomegranate juice, coconut water, and citrus juices. Stir well.

3. Place in the refrigerator and let chill for at least 3 to 4 hours.

4. Serve over ice in wine glasses, including the fruit.

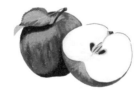

POMEGRANATE JUICE HAS THE HIGHEST ANTIOXIDANT PROFILE OF ANY JUICE, EVEN TRUMPING THE ANTIOXIDANT LEVELS IN RED WINE! WE TESTED OUR RECIPES WITH POM BRAND.

COS-NO-POLITAN

SERVES 2

The Cosmo is an iconic cocktail. Our mocktail version is equally sophisticated
and the perfect drink to sip at happy hour.

INGREDIENTS

1 cup coconut water

¼ cup orange juice

¼ cup cranberry juice (or diet cranberry juice or
tart cherry juice)

2 tablespoons lime juice

2 tablespoons lemon juice

Twist of lemon for garnish

TOOLS

Shaker

PREPARATION

1. Combine all the ingredients in a shaker and add ice.
   Shake vigorously for 30 seconds.

2. Strain the mixture into two martini glasses and garnish
   with a twist of lemon.

SINCE THIS RECIPE IS FLAVORED WITH FRESH FRUIT JUICES INSTEAD
OF CLEAR LIQUORS, THE COLOR WILL BE DIFFERENT, BUT THIS DRINK
CAPTURES THE FLAVORS OF THE CLASSIC COCKTAIL.

A "TWIST" IS A PIECE OF CITRUS ZEST USED TO GARNISH A COCKTAIL. YOU
CAN USE A KNIFE OR VEGETABLE PEELER TO TAKE OFF A WIDE PIECE OF
LEMON ZEST. TRY TO AVOID INCLUDING TOO MUCH OF THE PITH (THE
WHITE PART OF THE RIND), AS THIS IS QUITE BITTER.

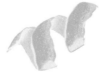

HORCHATA

Horchata is a sweet, creamy beverage. While different versions of horchata can be found around the world, our recipe was inspired by the rice-based variation, which you might encounter in the U.S. and Mexico. Sweetened with dates and a hint of cinnamon, our plant-based horchata makes for a refreshing drink or dessert!

INGREDIENTS

5 cups non-dairy milk

3 cups water

2 teaspoons vanilla extract

1 ⅓ cups long-grain brown rice, uncooked

6 pitted Medjool dates

1 teaspoon ground cinnamon

Cinnamon sticks for garnish

TOOLS

Blender

Strainer or nut milk bag

PREPARATION

1. Combine all the ingredients in a blender and blend until the rice is pulverized.

2. Place in the fridge and allow to soak for at least 4 hours.

3. Strain the mixture.

4. Fill four to six lowball or highball glasses with ice, depending on the desired serving size. Divide the strained horchata among the glasses.

5. Garnish with cinnamon sticks.

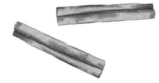

EASY BREEZY

Our take on the super simple Sea Breeze is equally easy to throw together and strikes the perfect balance between tart and sweet.

INGREDIENTS

2 ⅔ cups coconut water

1 ⅓ cups cranberry juice

½ cup grapefruit juice

¼ cup lime juice

Lime wheels or wedges for garnish

TOOLS

Pitcher

PREPARATION

1. Combine all the ingredients in a pitcher. Stir.

2. Divide the mixture among four lowball glasses.

3. Garnish with lime wheels or wedges.

SWAP THE CRANBERRY JUICE FOR PINEAPPLE JUICE TO MAKE A MOCKTAIL VERSION OF A BAY BREEZE—OR BETTER YET, MAKE A BLENDED VERSION WITH FROZEN PINEAPPLE!

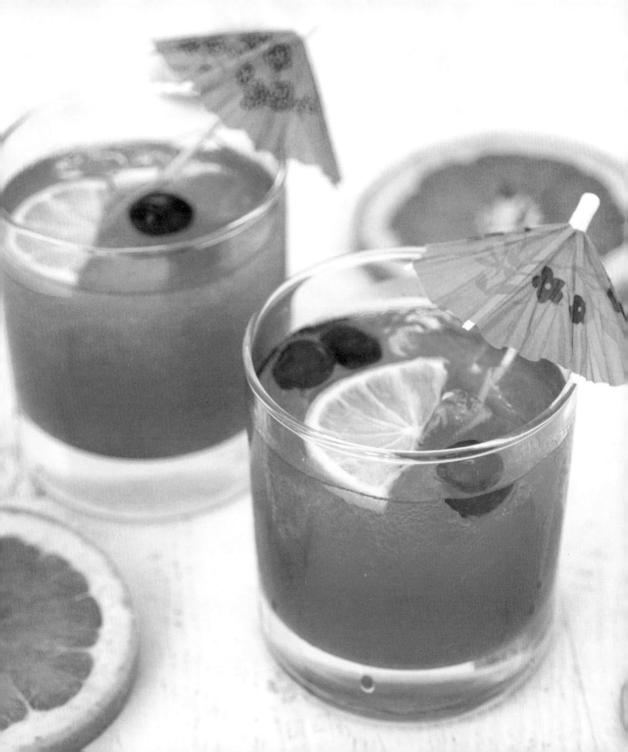

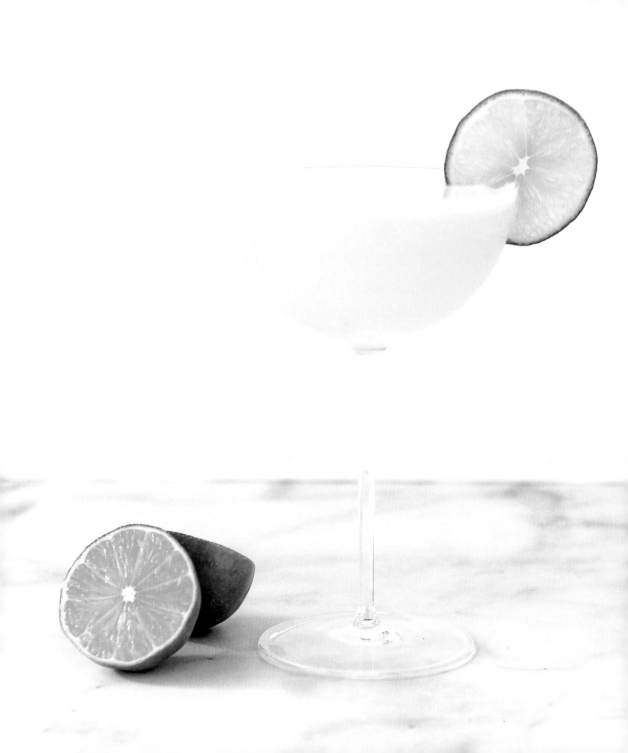

PISCO-LESS SOUR

SERVES 2

The Pisco Sour is typically made with fermented grape juice, lime juice, simple syrup, and egg whites. We adapted this Peruvian cocktail to be free of alcohol, added sugar, and eggs, while still delivering its classic foamy top and sour punch.

INGREDIENTS

⅔ cup white grape juice

⅔ cup coconut water

¼ cup and 2 tablespoons lime juice

1 tablespoon aquafaba

Lime wheels for garnish

TOOLS

Pitcher

PREPARATION

1. Combine all the ingredients in a pitcher. Stir.

2. Divide the mixture among two coupe or stemless wine glasses.

3. Garnish with lime wheels or wedges.

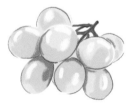

AQUAFABA IS THE LIQUID YOU SEE WHEN YOU OPEN A CAN OF CHICKPEAS. IT CAN BE USED AS A SUBSTITUTE FOR EGG WHITES IN COCKTAILS TO CREATE A FOAM EFFECT, AS WELL AS IN BAKING (E.G., TO MAKE MERINGUE). SIMPLY RESERVE SOME OF THE LIQUID BEFORE DRAINING THE CAN OF CHICKPEAS.

USE THE CHICKPEAS TO MAKE YOUR OWN HUMMUS, OR ADD TO A SALAD FOR PLANT-BASED PROTEIN.

CHAPTER

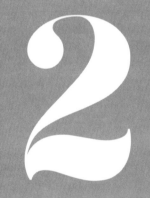

WITH A TWIST

We're taking it to the next level with these concoctions. In this section, we've crafted creative spins on traditional cocktail recipes, like a Watermelon Mock-jito and Blood Orange Mock-a-Rita, as well as unique drinks, like our Iced Orange Creamsicle and Cherry Licorice Soda.

COCONUT MOCK-JITO

A tropical spin on our classic Mock-jito recipe, this mocktail will transport you to paradise with every sip.

INGREDIENTS

20 mint leaves

2 tablespoons lime juice

2 teaspoons agave nectar

1 teaspoon apple cider vinegar

1 cup coconut water

2 tablespoons canned coconut milk

1 cup seltzer

Additional mint sprigs or leaves for garnish

TOOLS

Muddler

Shaker

PREPARATION

1. Muddle the mint leaves with the lime juice, agave nectar, and apple cider vinegar in the bottom of a shaker.

2. Add the coconut water, coconut milk, and ice.

3. Shake vigorously for 30 seconds.

4. Divide the shaken mixture between highball glasses.

5. Top with seltzer (½ cup per serving) and stir.

6. Garnish with mint.

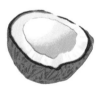

WE USE CANNED COCONUT MILK IN MANY OF OUR DESSERT MOCKTAIL RECIPES (SEE PAGE 80). STORE EXTRA COCONUT MILK IN AN AIRTIGHT CONTAINER FOR 4 TO 6 DAYS FOR LATER USE.

AS PHOTOGRAPHED, YOU CAN ADD A RIM OF DRIED COCONUT USING LIME JUICE TO WET THE GLASS. TOAST THE COCONUT AHEAD OF TIME TO ADD EVEN MORE FLAVOR!

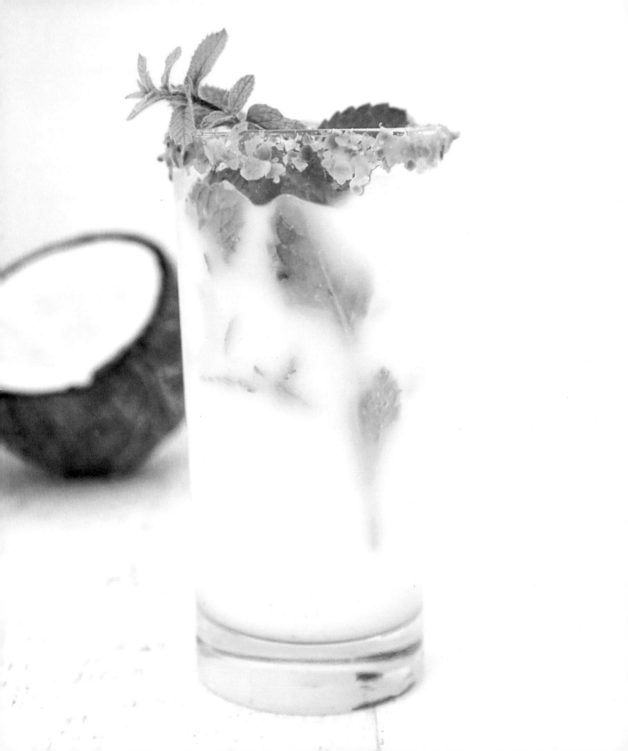

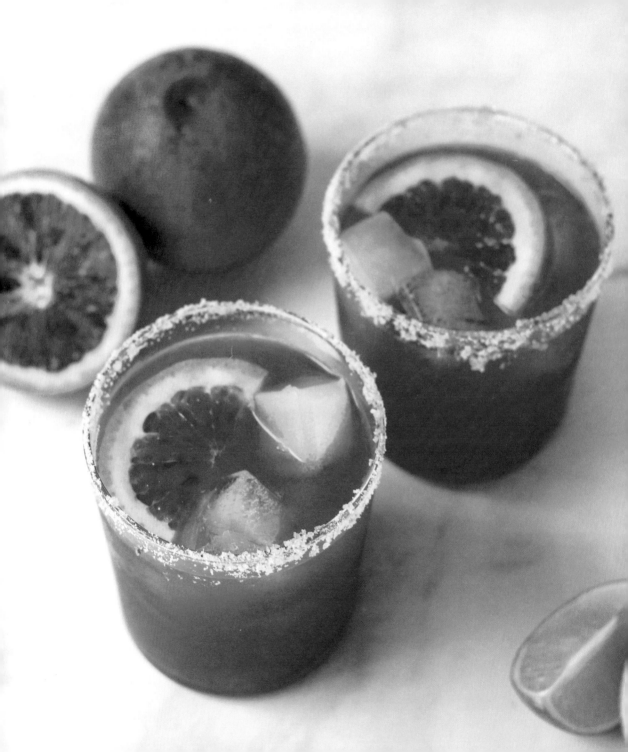

BLOOD ORANGE MOCK-A-RITA

Who says you can't enjoy a Mock-a-rita any time of the year? The addition of blood orange juice transforms this classic drink into a wintery mocktail. Plus, the vibrant color is to die for!

INGREDIENTS

SALTED RIM
Lime wedges
Sea salt

DRINK
1 cup coconut water
½ cup blood orange juice
¼ cup and 2 tablespoons lime juice
2 teaspoons agave nectar
Dash of salt

Blood orange slices for garnish

TOOLS
Shaker

PREPARATION

1. Rim two margarita or lowball glasses with salt (see page 10).
2. Combine all the ingredients in a shaker and add ice.
3. Shake vigorously.
4. Fill the rimmed glasses with ice and strain the shaken mixture into the glasses.
5. Garnish with blood orange slices.

IF YOU HAVE TROUBLE FINDING BLOOD ORANGES, YOU CAN SWAP IN YOUR FAVORITE CITRUS FRUIT.

BEE STING MOCK-A-RITA

SERVES 2

If you love a spicy Margarita, then this is the mocktail for you. The jalapeño
gives our Bee Sting Mock-a-rita quite the kick!

INGREDIENTS

SALTED RIM

Lime wedges

Sea salt

DRINK

3 to 4 slices fresh jalapeño (seeds removed if
you want to tone down the heat)

¼ cup lime juice

2 teaspoons honey or maple syrup

1 teaspoon apple cider vinegar

1 ⅓ cups maple or coconut water

Couple dashes of salt

Jalapeño slices and lime wedges for garnish

TOOLS

Muddler

Shaker

PREPARATION

1. Rim two margarita or lowball glasses with salt
   (see page 10).

2. Muddle the jalapeño, lime juice, honey, and apple cider
   vinegar in the bottom of a shaker.

3. Add the maple water and a sprinkle of salt.

4. Add ice and shake vigorously for 30 seconds.

5. Fill the rimmed glasses with ice and strain the shaken
   mixture into the glasses.

6. Garnish with jalapeño slices and lime wedges.

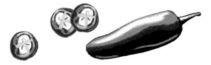

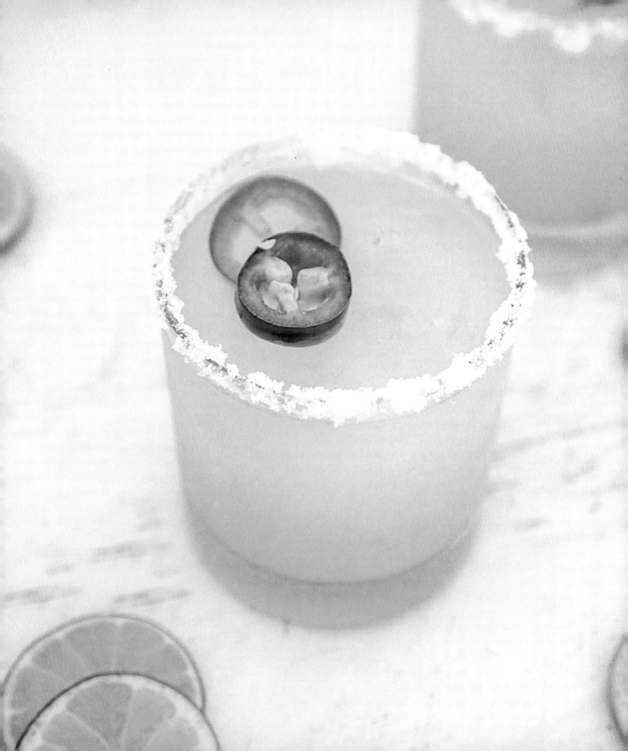

WATERMELON MOCK-JITO

SERVES 2

Watermelon pairs well with mint, so naturally, it makes a perfect addition to our Mock-jito! And because we use whole fruit, there is no need to add sweetener.

INGREDIENTS

1 ½ cups cubed watermelon

⅔ cup coconut water

20 mint leaves

2 tablespoons lime juice

1 teaspoon apple cider vinegar

⅔ cup seltzer

Additional mint sprigs or leaves for garnish

TOOLS

Blender

Muddler

Shaker

PREPARATION

1. Combine the watermelon cubes and coconut water in a blender and blend until smooth.

2. Muddle the mint leaves, lime juice, and apple cider vinegar in the bottom of a shaker.

3. Add the "watermelon water" and ice. Shake vigorously.

4. Divide the mixture between two highball glasses.

5. Top with seltzer (⅓ cup per serving) and stir.

6. Garnish with mint.

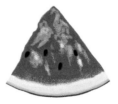

HONEY SAGE SOUR

SERVES 2

Sage adds a unique, savory element to this mocktail, which was inspired by a Whiskey Sour. Take it to the next level by adding aquafaba to create a foam effect!

INGREDIENTS

5 to 6 sage leaves

¼ cup lemon juice

2 teaspoons honey

1 teaspoon apple cider vinegar

1 ½ cups maple or coconut water

1 tablespoon aquafaba (optional)

Lemon peel for garnish

TOOLS

Muddler

Shaker

PREPARATION

1. Muddle the sage leaves, lemon juice, honey, and apple cider vinegar in the bottom of a shaker.

2. Add the coconut water to the shaker, along with the aquafaba, if using, and ice.

3. Shake vigorously for 30 seconds.

4. Fill two lowball glasses with ice and strain the shaken mixture into the glasses.

5. Garnish with lemon peel.

TO CREATE A FOAM EFFECT USING THE AQUAFABA, COMBINE ALL THE INGREDIENTS IN A SHAKER AND DRY SHAKE (WITHOUT ICE). THEN, SHAKE A SECOND TIME WITH ICE. SERVE.

USE EXTRA SAGE TO MAKE OUR APEROL-LESS SPRITZ OR WARM CIDER AND SAGE RECIPES ON PAGES 23 AND 151, RESPECTIVELY.

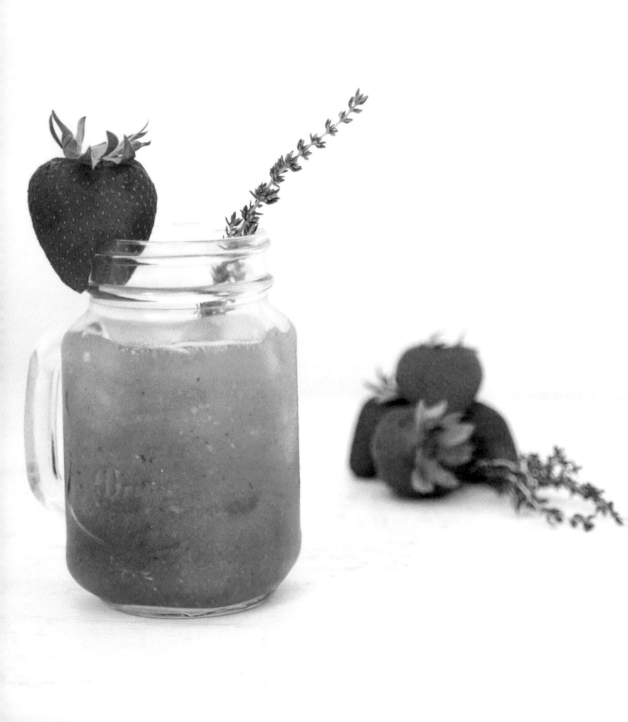

STRAWBERRY BALSAMIC SMASH

Slightly sweet, herbaceous, with a hint of acid: this mocktail has it all! It's so perfectly balanced and complex that you won't be able to stop sipping this drink.

INGREDIENTS

4 large, fresh strawberries, hulled and chopped

4 cucumber slices, quartered

2 sprigs fresh thyme

2 teaspoons honey

2 teaspoons balsamic vinegar

2 tablespoons lime juice

1 ½ cups coconut or maple water

Sliced strawberry, sliced cucumber, and thyme sprigs for garnish

TOOLS

Muddler

Shaker

PREPARATION

1. Muddle the strawberries, cucumber, and thyme in a shaker.

2. Add the honey, balsamic vinegar, and lime juice. Muddle again.

3. Add the coconut water and ice. Shake vigorously.

4. Strain the mixture into two lowball glasses.

5. Garnish with sprigs of thyme and strawberry or cucumber slices.

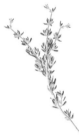

ENJOY LEFTOVER STRAWBERRIES IN A SALAD OR SMOOTHIE. OR BETTER YET, FREEZE THEM AND MAKE OUR TEQUILA-LESS SUNRISE ON PAGE 106.

BLACKBERRY MINT MOCKTAIL MULE

SERVES 2

This zesty and refreshing spin on the Moscow Mule uses fresh ginger instead of ginger beer. Made with berries and mint, this drink is perfect for any hot summer day.

INGREDIENTS

1 ⅓ cups coconut water

⅔ cup blackberries

2 teaspoons peeled and chopped fresh ginger

10 to 12 mint leaves

2 tablespoons lime juice

⅔ cup seltzer

Additional blackberries and mint leaves for garnish

TOOLS

Blender

Muddler

Shaker

PREPARATION

1. Combine the coconut water, blackberries, and ginger in a blender and blend until smooth.

2. Muddle the mint leaves and lime juice in the bottom of a shaker.

3. Add the blended mixture to the shaker along with ice. Shake vigorously.

4. Divide the shaken mixture between two copper mugs or highball glasses (option to strain). Top with ice as desired.

5. Top with seltzer (⅓ cup per serving).

6. Garnish with fresh blackberries and mint.

LEFTOVER GINGER? ADD IT TO A STIR-FRY, OR STEEP IN HOT WATER TO MAKE GINGER TEA.

YOU CAN SUBSTITUTE GINGER KOMBUCHA FOR THE FRESH GINGER AND COCONUT WATER, BUT DEPENDING ON THE KOMBUCHA, THE FLAVOR OF THE GINGER MAY NOT BE AS STRONG.

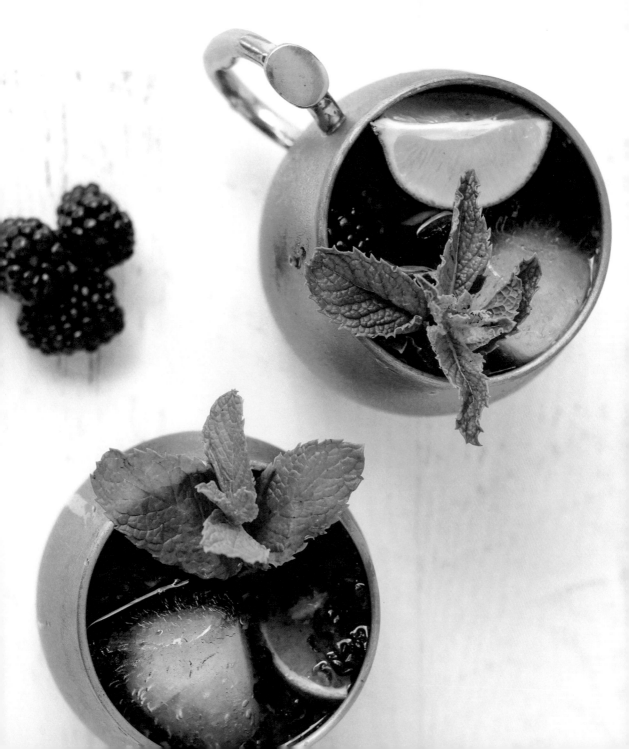

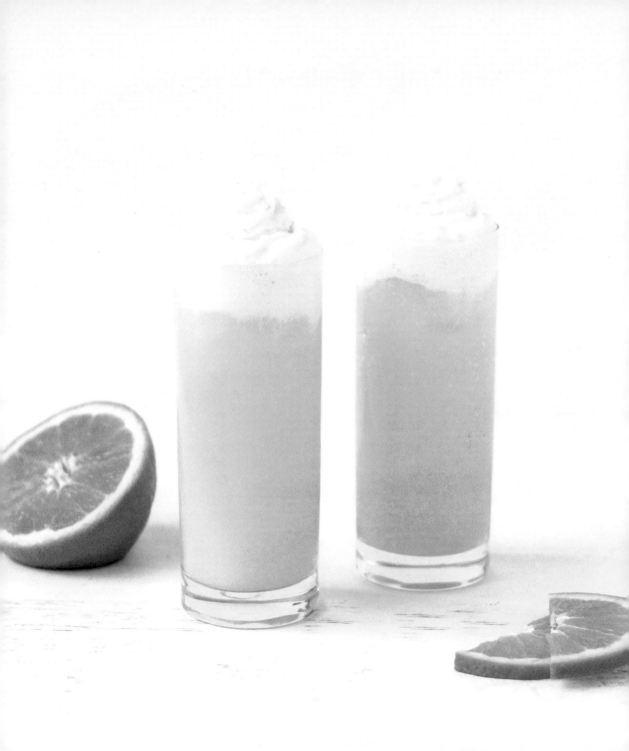

ICED ORANGE CREAMSICLE

SERVES **2**

Orange and vanilla are a match made in heaven. We combined them in this creamy but effervescent mocktail to capture the essence of your favorite childhood frozen treat!

INGREDIENTS

¼ cup canned coconut milk or cream

1 teaspoon agave nectar

½ teaspoon vanilla extract

1 cup orange juice

1 cup seltzer

Orange slices for garnish

Non-dairy whipped cream for topping

TOOLS

Shaker

PREPARATION

1. Combine the coconut milk, agave nectar, and vanilla extract in a shaker. Stir.

2. Add the orange juice and ice. Shake vigorously.

3. Fill two highball glasses with ice and strain the shaken mixture into the glasses.

4. Top with seltzer (½ cup per serving).

5. Garnish with orange slices and top with whipped cream.

CHERRY LICORICE SODA

SERVES 2

If you love licorice, then this is the drink for you! And if you don't, you should still give it a try. This mocktail has a unique flavor that will keep you coming back for more.

INGREDIENTS

1 cup pitted sweet cherries, fresh or frozen

2 teaspoons chopped tarragon leaves, loosely packed

1 cup coconut water

2 tablespoons lemon juice

⅔ cup seltzer

Tarragon sprigs for garnish

TOOLS

Blender

PREPARATION

1. Combine the cherries, tarragon leaves, coconut water, and lemon juice in a blender and blend until smooth.

2. Fill two highball glasses with ice and divide the blended mixture between the glasses.

3. Top with seltzer (⅓ cup per serving).

4. Garnish each glass with a spring of fresh tarragon.

USE EXTRA TARRAGON TO MAKE OUR CAROTENE COOLER (PAGE 134) IN THE DRINKS WITH BENEFITS SECTION.

YOU MAY NOTICE A REACTION BETWEEN THE FIBERS IN THE CHERRY AND THE CARBONATED WATER. SIMPLY STIR YOUR DRINK AND EVERYTHING WILL COME TOGETHER.

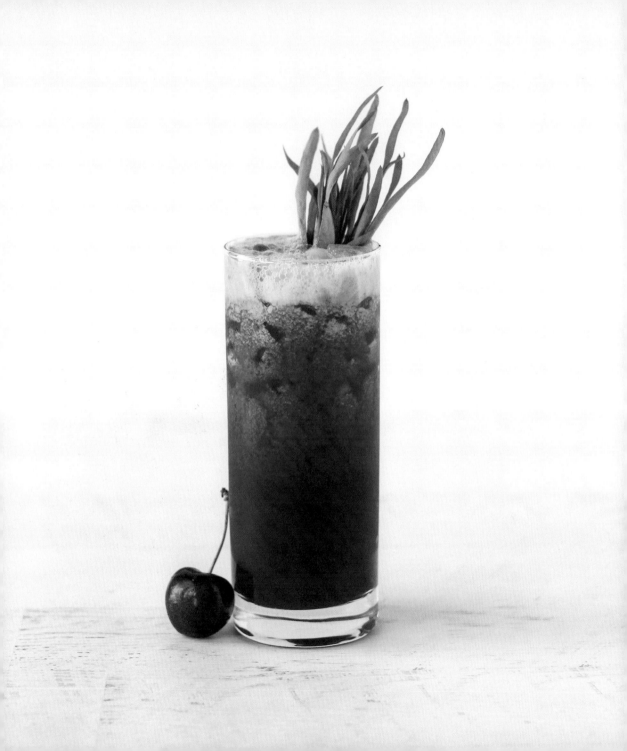

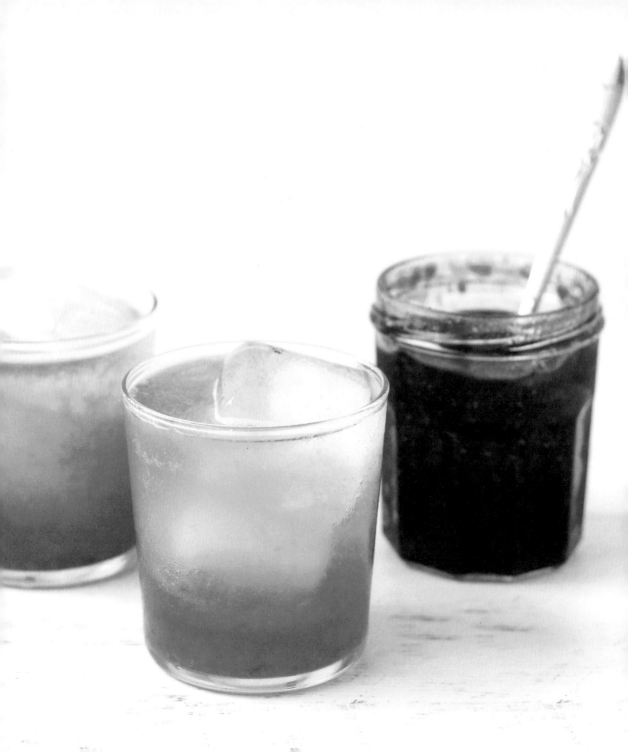

SUMMER JAM FRESCA

SERVES 2

Don't have fresh or frozen fruit around the house? No problem! You can use homemade or store-bought jam to add fruit flavor, sweetness, and texture to a mocktail. Shake up your mocktail routine with this easy and customizable recipe.

INGREDIENTS

1 cup coconut water

2 tablespoons lemon or lime juice

2 tablespoons high-quality jam (can be homemade or store-bought)

½ teaspoon apple cider vinegar

1 cup seltzer

Fresh herbs and fruit for garnish (see suggestions in the notes below)

TOOLS

Shaker

PREPARATION

1. Combine all the ingredients except the seltzer in a shaker.

2. Shake vigorously for 30 seconds.

3. Fill two lowball glasses with ice and strain the shaken mixture into the glasses.

4. Top with seltzer (½ cup per serving).

5. Garnish with fresh fruit and herbs.

SUGGESTED FLAVOR COMBINATIONS:

• STRAWBERRY JAM WITH LEMON JUICE AND MINT
• BLUEBERRY JAM WITH LEMON JUICE AND BASIL
• PEACH OR APRICOT JAM WITH LEMON JUICE AND THYME
• RASPBERRY JAM WITH LIME JUICE AND MINT
• CHERRY JAM WITH LIME JUICE AND TARRAGON
• BLACKBERRY JAM WITH LIME JUICE AND SAGE

TRY MAKING YOUR OWN JAM USING CHIA SEEDS FOR ADDED FIBER AND OMEGA-3s!

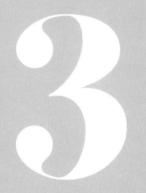

CHAPTER

3

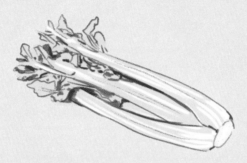

BRUNCH

*Make your next Sunday Funday truly
memorable with these lively mocktails.
From staple brunch beverages like our take
on the Mimosa and Bloody Mary, to more
playful drinks like our Pain-Free Pineapple
and Raspberry Float, we have a drink that
will please any crowd.*

GING-OSA

Missing your Mimosa at brunch? We've got you covered. Our mocktail version has fresh ginger and apple cider vinegar for an "alcoholic" bite.

INGREDIENTS

1 ½ cups orange juice

1 tablespoon and 1 teaspoon peeled and chopped fresh ginger

1 teaspoon apple cider vinegar

1 ½ cups seltzer

Orange slices and fresh thyme for garnish

TOOLS

Blender

Shaker

Pitcher

PREPARATION

1. Combine the orange juice, ginger, and apple cider vinegar in a blender and blend until the ginger pieces are imperceptible.

2. Pour the mixture into a shaker filled with ice. Shake vigorously.

3. Strain the shaken mixture into a pitcher and stir. Add the seltzer.

4. Divide the drink between four champagne glasses.

5. Garnish with orange slices and fresh thyme.

FOR A FUN VARIATION, SUBSTITUTE GRAPEFRUIT OR BLOOD ORANGE JUICE FOR THE ORANGE JUICE.

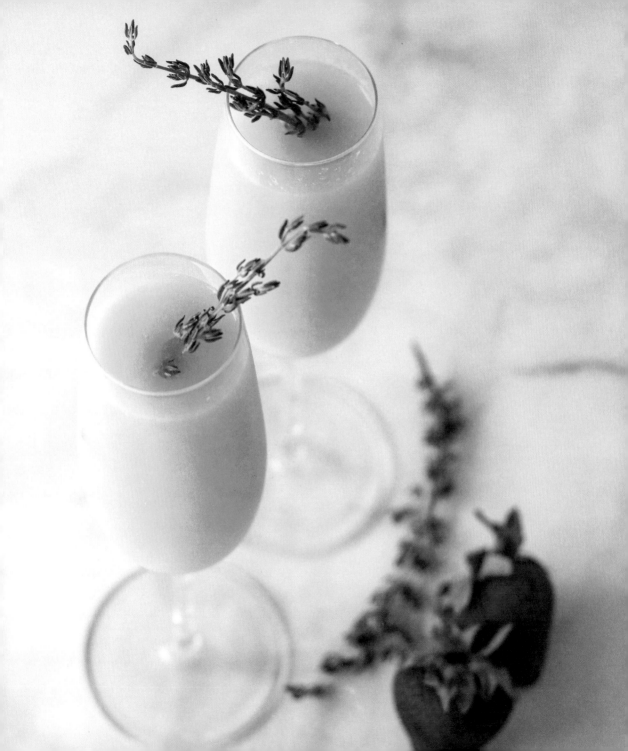

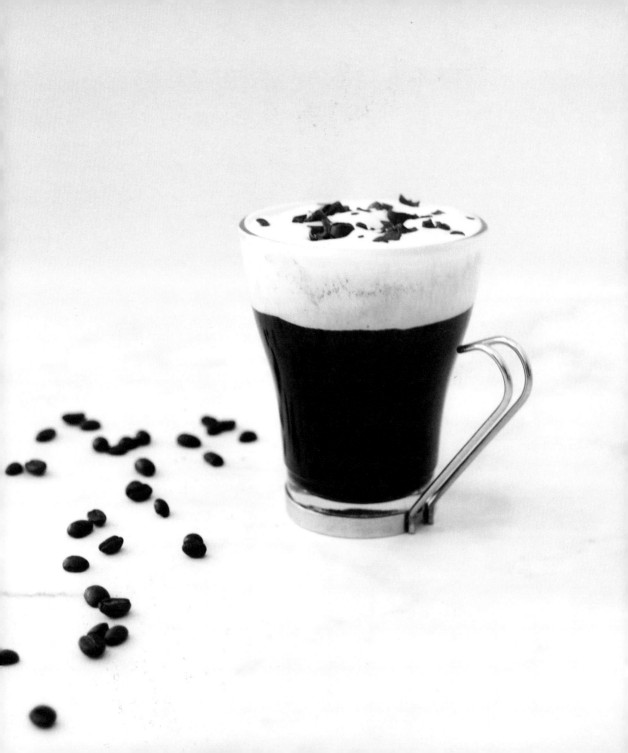

IR-ISH COFFEE

This mocktail is inspired by classic Irish Coffee, which is hot coffee mixed with Irish whiskey and sugar and topped with whipped cream.

INGREDIENTS

WHIPPED TOPPING

1 14-ounce can full-fat coconut milk

Maple syrup (to taste, starting with 1 tablespoon)

¼ teaspoon vanilla extract

COFFEE BASE

1 ⅓ cups strong brewed coffee

2 teaspoons agave nectar

½ teaspoon rum extract (optional)

¼ teaspoon vanilla extract

Cocoa powder for garnish

TOOLS

Hand mixer or whisk

Pitcher

PREPARATION

TO MAKE THE COCONUT WHIPPED TOPPING

1. Refrigerate a can of coconut milk overnight.

2. Scrape off the top layer of solidified coconut milk into a bowl. Whip the coconut milk solids together with the maple syrup and vanilla extract in a small mixing bowl with an electric mixer or a whisk for several minutes, until fluffy.

TO MAKE THE COFFEE BASE

1. In a pitcher, stir the hot coffee together with the agave nectar, rum extract, if using, and vanilla extract.

2. Divide the mixture between two mugs.

3. Top the coffee with the coconut whipped topping.

4. Garnish with cocoa powder.

FUN FACT:
LIGHT-ROAST COFFEE BEANS HAVE MORE CAFFEINE BY VOLUME THAN DARKER ROASTS!

BLUEBERRY BASIL COOLER

This unique mocktail looks pretty and is packed with flavor. Oh, and did we mention that it's nutritious as well? Blueberries are loaded with antioxidants and fiber, making this drink a winner on all fronts.

INGREDIENTS

½ cup frozen blueberries (or fresh blueberries)

6 large basil leaves

2 tablespoons lime juice

¼ cup white grape juice

1 cup coconut water

1 cup seltzer

Blueberries and basil leaves for garnish

TOOLS

Muddler

Shaker

PREPARATION

1. Gently muddle the blueberries, basil, and lime juice in the bottom of a shaker.

2. Add the grape juice, coconut water, and ice.

3. Shake vigorously for 30 seconds.

4. Divide the shaken mixture, including the ice, between two highball glasses, or strain into the glasses if desired.

5. Top with seltzer (½ cup per serving).

6. Garnish with basil leaves and fresh blueberries.

USE LEFTOVER BASIL TO MAKE HOMEMADE TOMATO SAUCE OR PESTO, OR ADD IT TO A SALAD.

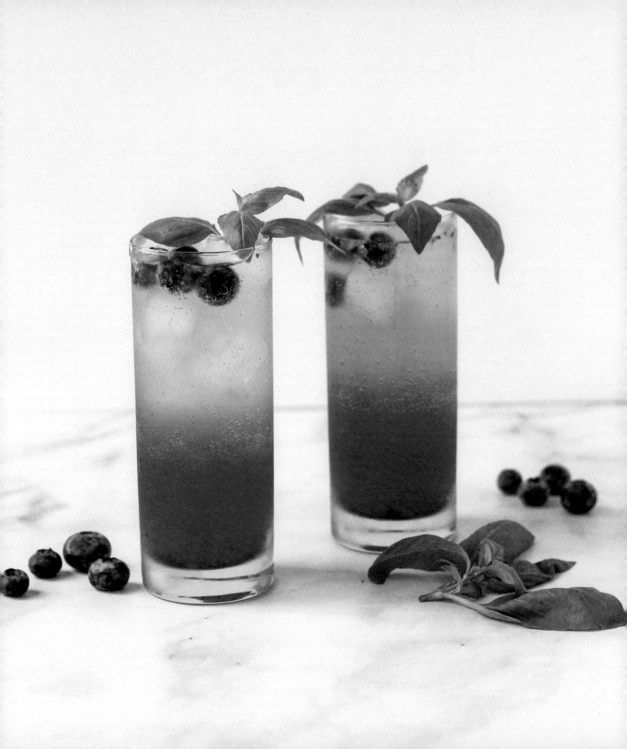

NO-BULL BLOODY

Transform your Virgin Mary with the addition of umami in the form of broth or stock. Based on the Bloody Bull, this mocktail is unique and ultra-savory.

INGREDIENTS

3 cups prepared tomato juice or vegetable juice (use low-sodium juice to control the amount of salt)

1 cup vegetable broth (homemade or store-bought)

2 tablespoons lime juice

2 tablespoons lemon juice

2 teaspoons prepared horseradish, or to taste

1 teaspoon hot sauce, or to taste (depending on the heat of your hot sauce)

½ teaspoon Worcestershire sauce

Salt (or seasoned salt) to taste

½ teaspoon ground black pepper

½ teaspoon smoked paprika

Celery sticks for garnish

TOOLS

Pitcher

PREPARATION

1. Combine all the ingredients in a pitcher and stir.

2. Chill for a few hours or overnight. The longer this drink sits, the more the flavors will develop.

3. Fill four highball glasses with ice and divide the mixture among the glasses.

4. Garnish with celery sticks.

SOOTHING SPRITZER

Enjoy a relaxing morning with this brunch beverage. Made with homemade
lavender syrup, this soothing drink will melt your worries away. If you prefer,
you can also purchase prepared lavender syrup.

INGREDIENTS

LAVENDER SYRUP

¼ cup honey

¼ cup water

1 teaspoon culinary lavender

DRINK

½ cup fresh or frozen blueberries

2 tablespoons lavender syrup

1 cup coconut water

2 tablespoons lemon juice

1 teaspoon apple cider vinegar

1 cup seltzer

Lemon peel for garnish

TOOLS

Muddler

Saucepan

Strainer or nut milk bag

PREPARATION

TO MAKE THE LAVENDER SYRUP

1. Combine the honey, water, and lavender in a saucepan over medium heat.

2. When the mixture comes to a boil, simmer for a minute, then take off the heat and allow to cool.

3. Let the mixture steep for 10 minutes.

4. Strain out the lavender and store the syrup in the fridge.

TO MAKE THE DRINK

1. Divide the blueberries between two highball glasses and add 1 tablespoon of lavender syrup to each glass. Muddle.

2. Divide the coconut water, lemon juice, and apple cider vinegar between each glass.

3. Add ice and top with seltzer (½ cup per serving).

4. Garnish with lemon peel.

MAKE SURE YOU USE LAVENDER THAT IS SAFE FOR
CONSUMPTION ("CULINARY" LAVENDER).

TO INCREASE THE LAVENDER FLAVOR IN YOUR
DRINKS, PREPARE THE LAVENDER SYRUP WITH UP
TO 1 TABLESPOON OF CULINARY LAVENDER.

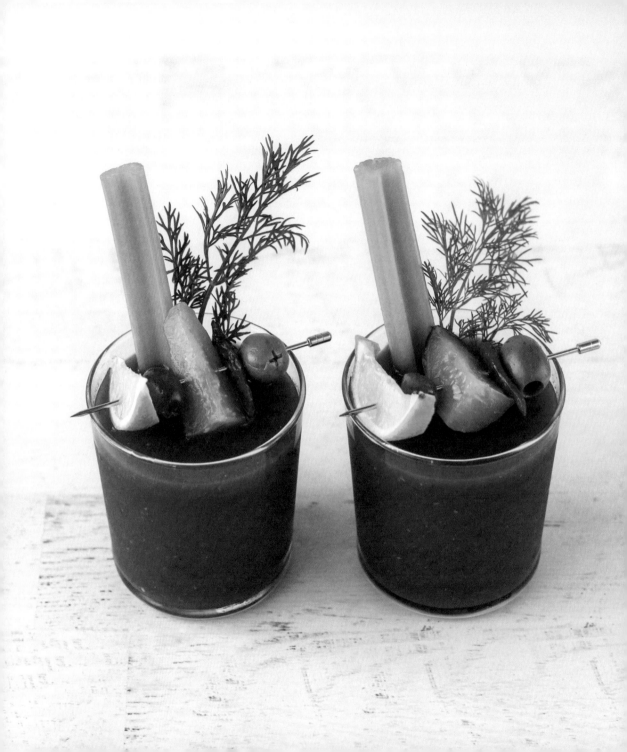

PICKLED MARY

SERVES 4-6

We love the addition of pickle juice to a classic Bloody Mary, so we decided to take it to the next level. Capers add salt and brine, while dill adds freshness and an herbaceous note.

INGREDIENTS

4 cups prepared tomato juice or vegetable juice (we use low-sodium so we can control the amount of salt)

½ cup and 2 tablespoons dill pickle juice

¼ cup lemon juice

2 teaspoons prepared horseradish, or to taste

2 teaspoons hot sauce, or to taste (may need to adjust based on what type of hot sauce you have on hand!)

1 teaspoon Worcestershire sauce

¼ cup chopped fresh dill

1 tablespoon and 1 teaspoon capers

½ to 1 teaspoon ground black pepper, to taste

Celery salt, seasoned salt, or regular salt to taste

Celery sticks, lemon wedges, and dill for garnish

TOOLS

Pitcher

PREPARATION

1. Combine all the ingredients in a pitcher. Stir to mix.

2. Chill for a few hours or overnight. The longer this drink sits, the more the flavors will develop.

3. Fill highball glasses with ice and divide the mixture among the glasses.

4. Garnish with celery, lemon wedges, or dill.

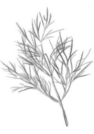

PLAY AROUND WITH THE HORSERADISH, HOT SAUCE, AND BLACK PEPPER QUANTITIES TO MAKE THIS VERSION OF A BLOODY MARY PERFECT FOR YOU.

DILL CAN ADD FLAVOR TO A CHICKPEA SALAD.

SPICED VANILLA PEAR BELLINI

With warming spices and vanilla, this is the perfect mocktail to serve at your holiday brunch!

INGREDIENTS

1 cup chopped pear

1 cup coconut water

1 tablespoon and 1 teaspoon lemon juice

1 tablespoon and 1 teaspoon vanilla extract

1 teaspoon apple cider vinegar

¼ teaspoon ground cinnamon

Few shakes ground cardamom

1 ⅓ cups seltzer

TOOLS

Blender

Strainer or nut milk bag (optional)

PREPARATION

1. Combine all the ingredients except the seltzer in a blender and blend until smooth.

2. Strain the mixture, if desired, then divide among four champagne glasses.

3. Top with seltzer (⅓ cup per serving).

YOU MAY NOTICE A REACTION BETWEEN THE FIBERS IN THE PEAR AND THE CARBONATED WATER. GIVE THE DRINK A STIR, AND IT WILL COME TOGETHER.

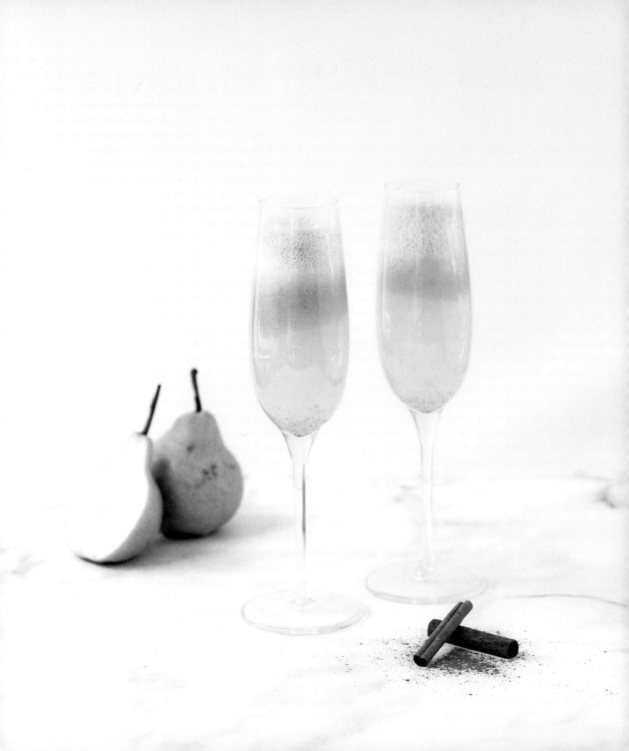

JUST PEACHY MOCKTAIL

SERVES 4

We transformed a classic '80s cocktail, the Fuzzy Navel, into a lightly-sweet, nutrient-dense mocktail made with whole fruit instead of peach schnapps.

INGREDIENTS

12 to 16 slices frozen peach (approximately 1 ⅓ to 1 ½ cups sliced peach)

2 cups coconut water

1 ⅓ cups orange juice

1 teaspoon apple cider vinegar

TOOLS

Blender

PREPARATION

1. Combine all the ingredients in a blender and blend until frothy.

2. Divide the blended mixture among four lowball glasses.

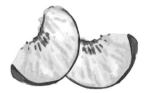

GOLDEN MILK ELIXIR

Our take on the trendy Golden Milk Latte is rich and comforting. Start (or end) your day with this sunny, spicy, and warming beverage.

INGREDIENTS

2 ½ cups non-dairy milk

¼ cup canned coconut milk

1 tablespoon and 1 teaspoon sweetener of choice

½ teaspoon vanilla extract

1 teaspoon ground turmeric

½ teaspoon ground cinnamon

½ teaspoon ground ginger

Couple pinches ground black pepper

Couple pinches ground cardamom

Cinnamon sticks for garnish

TOOLS

Saucepan

PREPARATION

1. Combine all the ingredients in a saucepan over medium heat and heat slowly, whisking to incorporate the spices. Do not let the mixture boil.

2. Divide the mixture between two mugs.

3. Garnish with cinnamon sticks.

THIS DRINK IS ALSO DELICIOUS SERVED OVER ICE!

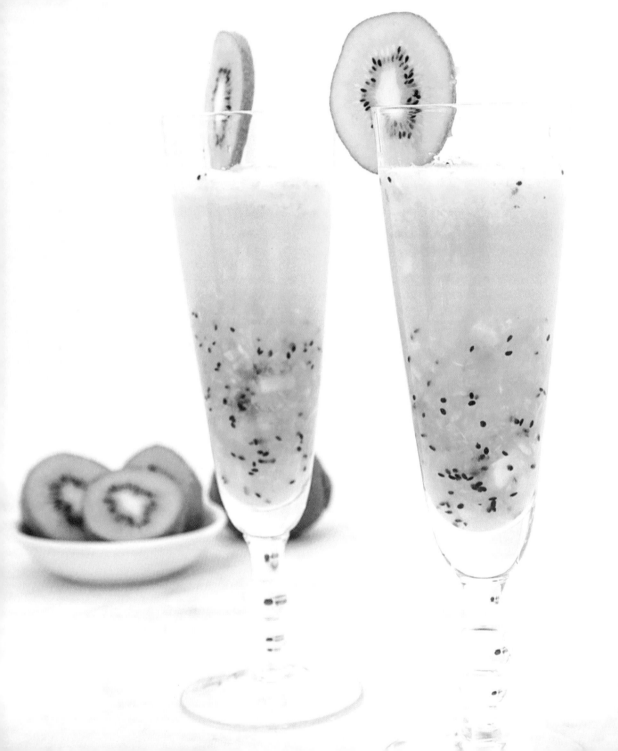

KIWI NO-SECCO

Prosecco just got a fruity makeover. This colorful, bubbly mocktail packs a vitamin C punch.

INGREDIENTS

½ cup peeled and chopped kiwi

1 teaspoon peeled and chopped fresh ginger

½ cup coconut water

3 tablespoons white grape juice

1 tablespoon lemon juice

½ to ⅔ cup seltzer

Extra kiwi for garnish

TOOLS

Blender

Shaker

Strainer or nut milk bag

PREPARATION

1. Combine the kiwi, ginger, coconut water, grape juice, and lemon juice in a blender and blend on high for one minute.

2. Strain the mixture into a shaker and add ice. Shake vigorously.

3. Divide the shaken mixture between two champagne glasses.

4. Top with seltzer (¼-⅓ cup per serving).

5. Garnish with kiwi slices.

DID YOU KNOW THE SKIN OF THE KIWI IS COMPLETELY EDIBLE? NEXT TIME YOU EAT A KIWI, GIVE IT A TRY FOR AN EXTRA NUTRIENT BOOST.

PAIN-FREE PINEAPPLE

Ease your way into the day with this alcohol-free take on the Painkiller cocktail,
a classic and popular tiki drink.

INGREDIENTS

1 ⅓ cups fresh or frozen pineapple

2 cups coconut water

½ cup canned coconut milk

½ cup orange juice

2 teaspoons apple cider vinegar

Couple dashes ground nutmeg

Pineapple slices and ground nutmeg for garnish

TOOLS

Blender

PREPARATION

1. Combine all the ingredients in a blender and blend until smooth and frothy.

2. Fill four lowball glasses with ice and divide the blended mixture among the glasses.

3. Top with nutmeg and garnish with a pineapple wedge.

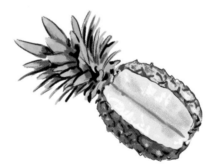

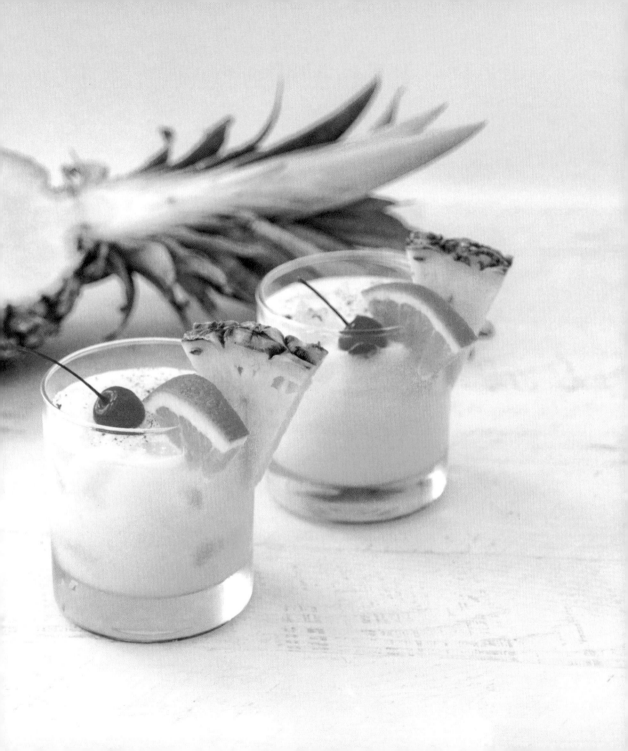

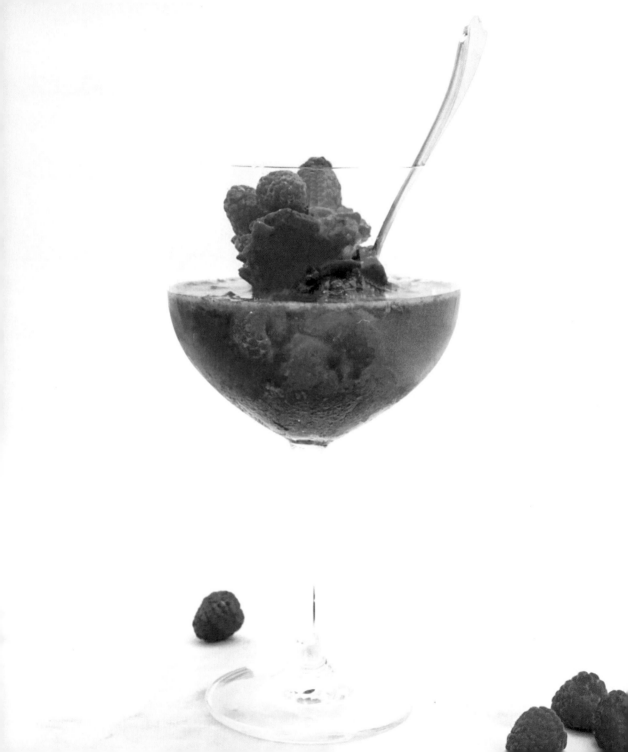

RASPBERRY SORBET FLOAT

Impress your friends with this classy beverage. This float looks like a dessert
but makes for an elegant brunch drink!

INGREDIENTS

INSTANT RASPBERRY SORBET

2 cups frozen raspberries

2 tablespoons agave nectar or honey

SPARKLING BEVERAGE

2 cups coconut water

¼ cup and 2 tablespoons white grape juice

¼ cup lemon juice

1 teaspoon apple cider vinegar

1 ⅓ cups seltzer

DON'T WANT TO MAKE YOUR OWN
SORBET? NO PROBLEM. WHEN
BUYING SORBET AT THE GROCERY
STORE, LOOK FOR BRANDS THAT
HAVE LOWER ADDED SUGAR
CONTENT. FEEL FREE TO SWAP
RASPBERRY FOR YOUR FAVORITE
FLAVOR! THE SPARKLING BEVERAGE
WOULD ALSO BE FUN TO SERVE
WITH A HOMEMADE OR STORE-
BOUGHT LOW-SUGAR POPSICLE.

TOOLS

Blender

Ice cream scoop or melon baller

Shaker

PREPARATION

TO MAKE THE RASPBERRY SORBET

1. Combine the frozen raspberries and sweetener in a blender and blend until smooth. Note: if using honey for the sweetener, be sure to add the raspberries to the blender first, followed by the honey.

TO MAKE THE SPARKLING BEVERAGE

1. Combine the coconut water, white grape juice, lemon juice, and apple cider vinegar in a shaker with ice. Shake well.

2. Strain the shaken mixture into four wine glasses or lowball glasses.

3. Scoop out the raspberry sorbet using a small ice cream scoop or melon baller and gently place a scoop into each filled glass.

4. Top with seltzer (⅓ cup per serving).

CHAPTER

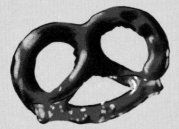

DESSERT

Made with whole fruits, and even vegetables, our dessert mock-tini drinks make for a quick and easy treat. You can enjoy these delicious mocktails after dinner or at any time of day!

CHOCOLATE MOUSSE MOCK-TINI

This Chocolate Mousse Mock-tini gets its decadent, creamy consistency from a secret ingredient: avocado! We promise you won't taste it.

INGREDIENTS

RIM

2 ounces dark chocolate, melted

DRINK

4 cups non-dairy milk

½ cup chopped avocado

3 ounces dark chocolate, melted

6 pitted Medjool dates

¼ cup unsweetened cocoa or cacao powder

2 teaspoons vanilla extract

TOOLS

Blender

PREPARATION

1. Rim four martini glasses by dipping them in the melted chocolate.

2. Place the glasses in the refrigerator for 10 minutes to allow the chocolate to harden.

3. Combine all the drink ingredients in a blender.

4. Blend on high until the dates are broken up for evenly distributed sweetness.

5. Divide the blended mixture among the chilled martini glasses.

CHOOSE DARK CHOCOLATE WITH GREATER THAN 70% COCOA FOR ADDED HEALTH BENEFITS LIKE FLAVONOIDS, IRON, AND MAGNESIUM—AND LOWER SUGAR CONTENT.

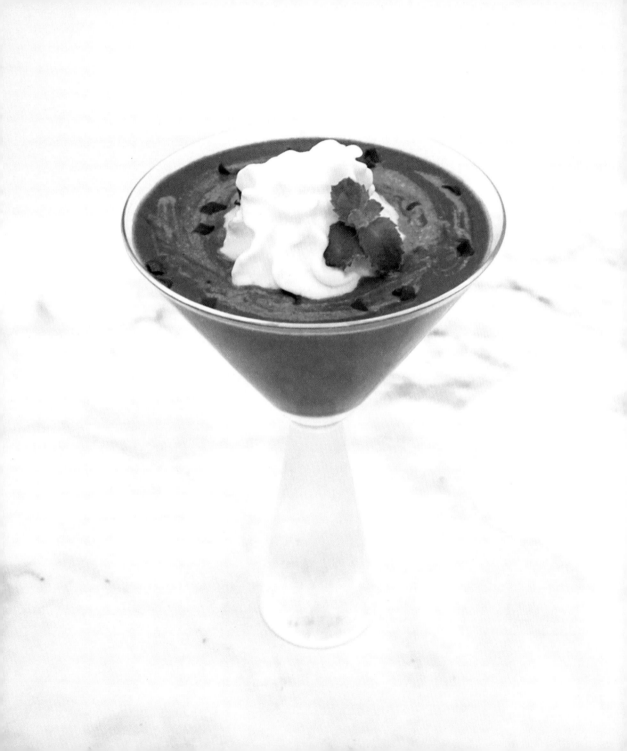

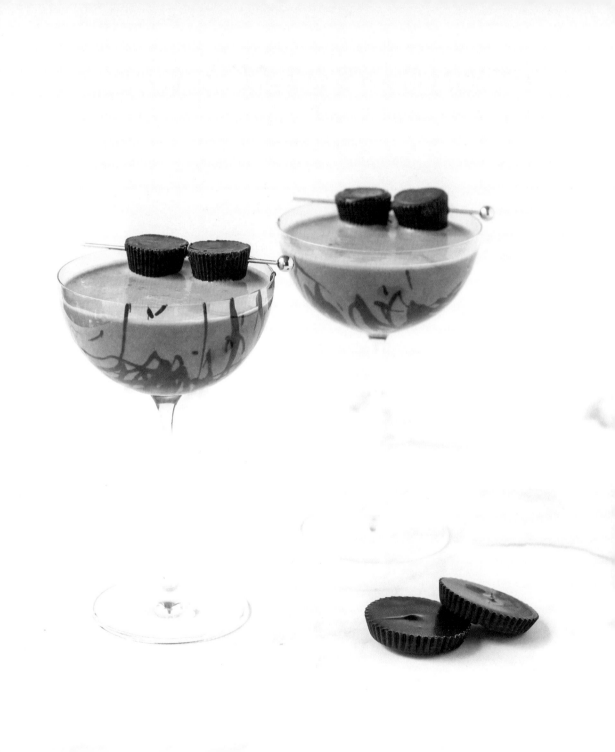

PEANUT BUTTER CUP
MOCK-TINI

Peanut butter and chocolate are a classic combination. This Mock-tini captures the essence of the beloved peanut butter cup, but it is sweetened with dates rather than added sugar.

INGREDIENTS

3 cups non-dairy milk

½ cup canned coconut milk

¼ cup peanut butter

¼ cup cocoa or cacao powder

8 pitted Medjool dates

Few dashes salt

Melted chocolate and peanut butter cups
for garnish

TOOLS

Blender

PREPARATION

1. Combine all the ingredients in a blender.

2. Blend on high until the dates are broken up for evenly distributed sweetness.

3. Divide the mixture among four chilled martini glasses.

4. Garnish with melted chocolate and peanut butter cups.

LOOK FOR NATURAL PEANUT BUTTER THAT CONTAINS NO ADDED
SUGAR OR OILS.

TIRAMISU MOCK-TINI

Craving an indulgent dessert? This Mock-tini has you covered. Creamy, chocolatey, and lightly sweet with a hint of coffee . . . what's not to love?

INGREDIENTS

1 cup non-dairy milk

¾ cup strong brewed coffee, chilled

¼ cup canned coconut milk

1 tablespoon and 1 teaspoon maple syrup

2 teaspoons cocoa or cacao powder

½ teaspoon vanilla

¼ teaspoon ground cinnamon

¼ teaspoon rum extract (optional)

Cocoa powder or chocolate shavings for garnish

TOOLS

Shaker

PREPARATION

1. Combine all the ingredients in a shaker filled with ice.

2. Shake vigorously for 30 seconds.

3. Strain the shaken mixture into two chilled martini glasses.

4. Garnish with cocoa powder or chocolate shavings.

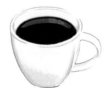

IT WOULD ALSO BE FUN TO SERVE THIS DESSERT MOCK-TINI WITH LADYFINGER COOKIES, WHICH ARE USED TO MAKE TIRAMISU.

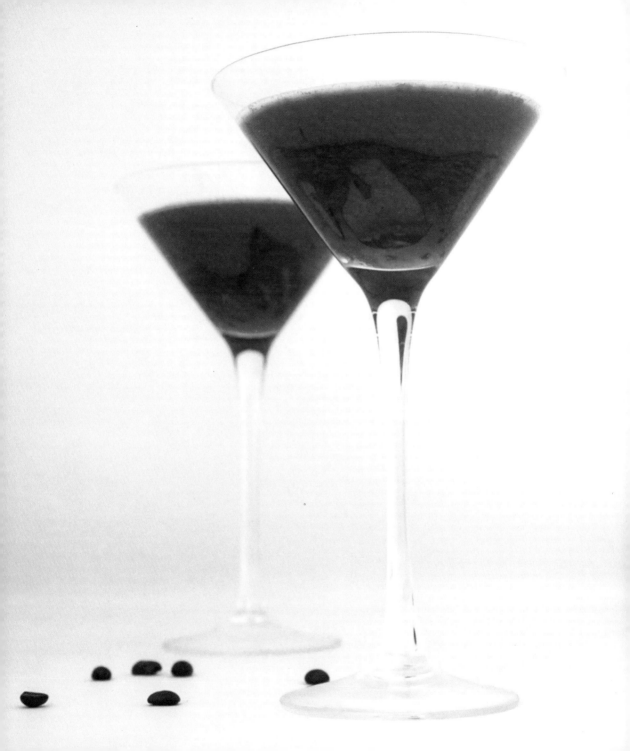

OATMEAL COOKIE MOCK-TINI

Have a hankering for a cookie but don't want to bake a whole batch? This Mock-tini is warmly spiced and packed with fiber in the form of oats and dates!

INGREDIENTS

3 cups oat milk

½ cup canned coconut milk

½ cup rolled oats

4 pitted Medjool dates

1 teaspoon vanilla extract

½ teaspoon ground cinnamon

4 dashes ground nutmeg

Couple dashes of salt

Additional ground cinnamon and oats for garnish

TOOLS

Blender

PREPARATION

1. Combine all the ingredients in a blender.

2. Blend on high until the dates are broken up for evenly distributed sweetness.

3. Divide the blended mixture among four chilled martini glasses.

4. Garnish with a sprinkle of ground cinnamon and oats.

PB&J MOCK-TINI

SERVES 4

This playful drink is a fun throwback to your favorite childhood treat, with a healthy, grown-up twist. Frozen cauliflower adds creaminess and nutrients (with no flavor), making this drink an easy way to get in your veggies.

INGREDIENTS

2 ⅔ cups non-dairy milk

1 cup frozen cauliflower or cauliflower rice (be sure to use plain!)

1 cup frozen blueberries or cherries

4 pitted Medjool dates

¼ cup peanut butter or nut butter of choice

Few shakes ground cinnamon

Couple shakes ground cardamom

Couple dashes salt

TOOLS

Blender

PREPARATION

1. Combine all the drink ingredients in a blender.

2. Blend on high until the dates are broken up for evenly distributed sweetness.

3. Divide the blended mixture among four chilled martini glasses.

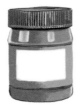

FOR A NUT-FREE VARIATION, SUBSTITUTE YOUR FAVORITE SEED BUTTER FOR THE PEANUT BUTTER.

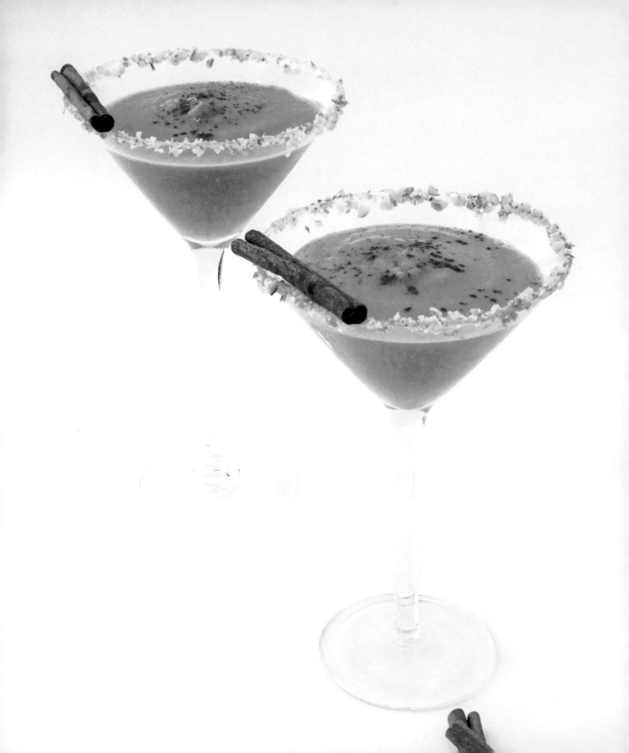

PUMPKIN PIE MOCK-TINI

SERVES 4

Our Pumpkin Pie Mock-tini is one of our favorite seasonal recipes, perfect for
Halloween and Thanksgiving parties!

INGREDIENTS

RIM

2 tablespoons chopped walnuts (or graham
crackers, for a nut-free version)

2 teaspoons maple syrup (plus more as needed)

DRINK

3 cups non-dairy milk

1 ⅓ cups canned pumpkin puree (avoid
pumpkin pie filling)

6 to 8 pitted Medjool dates

3 teaspoons pumpkin pie spice

1 teaspoon vanilla extract

Couple pinches salt

Coconut whipped cream and ground cinnamon
for garnish

TOOLS

Blender

PREPARATION

1. Rim four martini glasses by dipping them into the maple
   syrup, then into the chopped walnuts (see page 10).

2. Combine all the drink ingredients in a blender.

3. Blend on high until the dates are broken up for evenly
   distributed sweetness.

4. Divide the mixture among the prepared glasses.

5. Garnish each drink with a dollop of coconut whipped
   cream and a sprinkle of cinnamon.

EXTRA CANNED PUMPKIN?
USE IT TO MAKE PUMPKIN
BREAD OR COOKIES!

SALTED CARAMEL MOCK-TINI

This mocktail is decadence in a glass. Salty, sweet, and rich, it's like drinking a candy bar!

INGREDIENTS

SALTED DATE CARAMEL

8 pitted Medjool dates

½ cup non-dairy milk

¼ cup canned coconut milk

¼ teaspoon vanilla extract

¼ teaspoon salt

RIM

Date caramel and crushed salted pretzels or sea salt

DRINK

4 cups non-dairy milk

½ cup and 2 tablespoons date caramel (or more for extra caramel flavor)

½ cup canned coconut milk

2 teaspoons vanilla extract

Few shakes sea salt

Caramel candy or additional salted date caramel and salted pretzels for garnish

TOOLS

Blender

PREPARATION

TO MAKE THE DATE CARAMEL

1. Combine all the ingredients in a blender. Blend on high until the dates are broken up. Measure out at least ½ cup and 2 tablespoons and set aside for the drinks, then pour some of the remaining date caramel into a shallow bowl or plate.

TO PREPARE THE DRINK

1. Dip the rims of four martini glasses into the caramel, then into the crushed pretzels (see page 10).

2. Combine all the drink ingredients in the blender and blend on high until smooth.

3. Divide the mixture among the prepared martini glasses.

4. Garnish with extra caramel sauce, your favorite caramel candy, or salted pretzels.

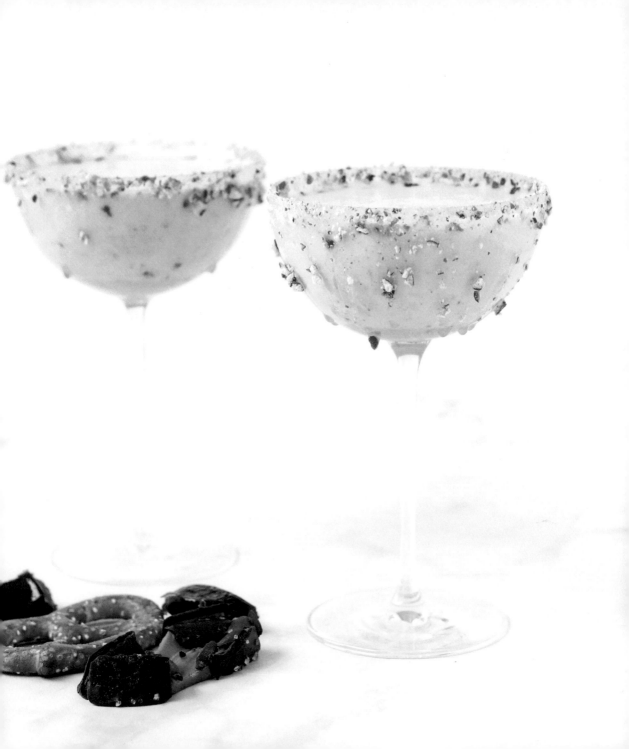

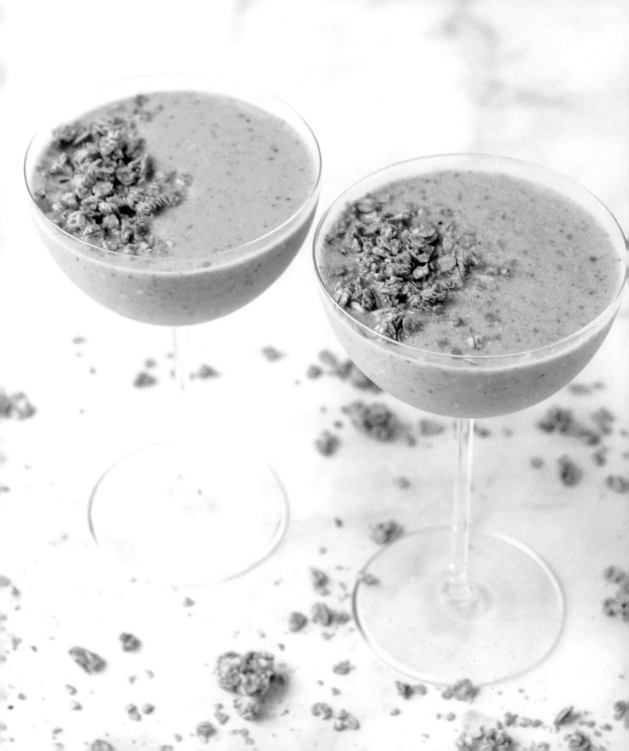

STRAWBERRY RHUBARB MOCK-TINI

Sweet strawberries paired with tart rhubarb blended up into a creamy dessert mocktail. Could there be a tastier way to eat your fruits and veggies?

INGREDIENTS

RIM

2 teaspoons maple syrup

2 tablespoons granola or crushed graham crackers

DRINK

2 ⅔ cups non-dairy milk

¼ cup canned coconut milk

2 cups frozen strawberries

1 cup chopped rhubarb

½ cup rolled oats

4 pitted Medjool dates

Ice cream or whipped cream for garnish

TOOLS

Blender

PREPARATION

1. Rim four martini glasses by dipping them into the maple syrup, then into the granola or graham crackers.

2. Combine all the drink ingredients in a blender and blend until smooth.

3. Divide the blended mixture among the prepared martini glasses.

4. Top with whipped cream or vanilla ice cream.

NO RHUBARB AVAILABLE? THIS DRINK IS STILL PERFECTLY DELICIOUS WITHOUT IT—IT TASTES LIKE A STRAWBERRIES AND CREAM SHAKE!

LEMON BAR MOCK-TINI

We transformed this beloved classic treat into a bright and citrusy mocktail.
We used rolled oats to capture the essence of a shortbread crust, and freshly
squeezed lemon juice and dates for the sweet and tangy filling.

INGREDIENTS

RIM

2 teaspoons lemon juice or maple syrup

2 tablespoons finely ground graham crackers or
walnuts

DRINK

2 ⅔ cups non-dairy milk

1 ⅓ cups frozen pineapple

¾ cup lemon juice

4 pitted Medjool dates

¼ cup rolled oats

2 teaspoons vanilla extract

Coconut whipped cream and lemon slices
for garnish

TOOLS

Blender

PREPARATION

1. Rim four martini glasses by wetting with the lemon juice
   or maple syrup, then dipping into the crushed graham
   crackers or walnuts (see page 10).

2. Combine all the drink ingredients in a blender.

3. Blend on high until the dates are broken up for evenly
   distributed sweetness.

4. Divide the blended mixture among the prepared
   martini glasses.

5. Garnish with a dollop of coconut whipped cream and
   lemon slices.

SAVE EXTRA FROZEN PINEAPPLE FOR ANOTHER MOCKTAIL.
LIKE THE PIÑA COL-NADA!

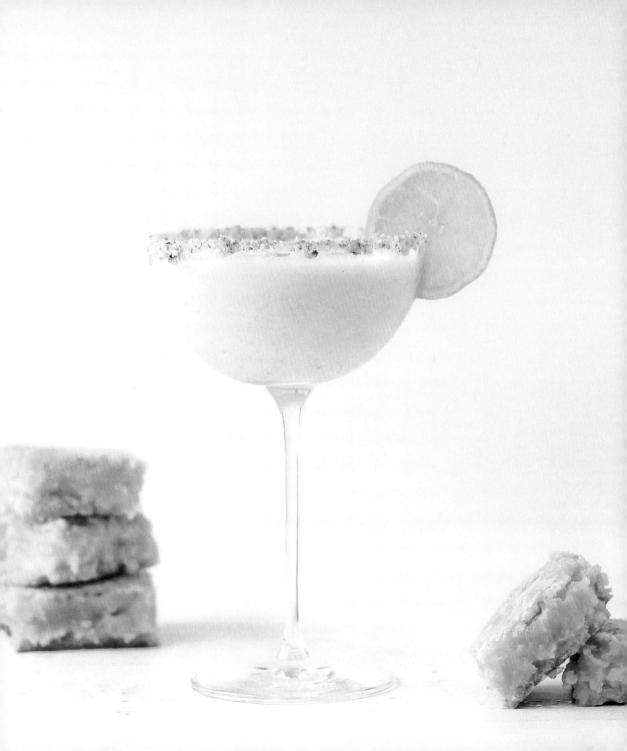

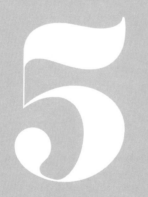

CHAPTER

5

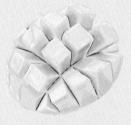

FROZEN

From classic frozen cocktails like the Piña Colada to trendy treats like Frosé, we've got alcohol-free, nutrient-dense recipes that are perfect by the pool, or whenever you need a getaway!

PIÑA COL-NADA

"If you like Piña Coladas . . ." but not the sugar and rum, one sip of our Piña Col-nada and you will instantly feel like you're on vacation.

INGREDIENTS

4 cups frozen pineapple

1 cup frozen cauliflower or cauliflower rice

2 cups unsweetened coconut milk (from a carton)

½ cup canned coconut milk

Couple squeezes of fresh lime juice

Pineapple, orange slices, or maraschino cherries for garnish

TOOLS

Blender

PREPARATION

1. Combine all the drink ingredients in a blender.

2. Blend on high until well combined.

3. Divide the mixture among margarita or hurricane glasses.

4. Garnish with pineapple, orange slices, or maraschino cherries.

FROZEN CAULIFLOWER HELPS TO MAKE THIS DRINK EXTRA CREAMY AND NUTRITIOUS WITHOUT AFFECTING THE FLAVOR.

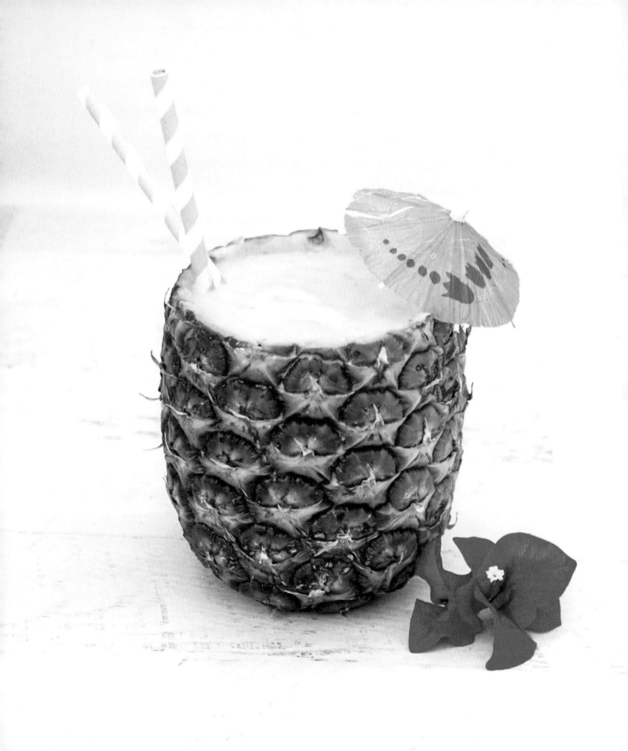

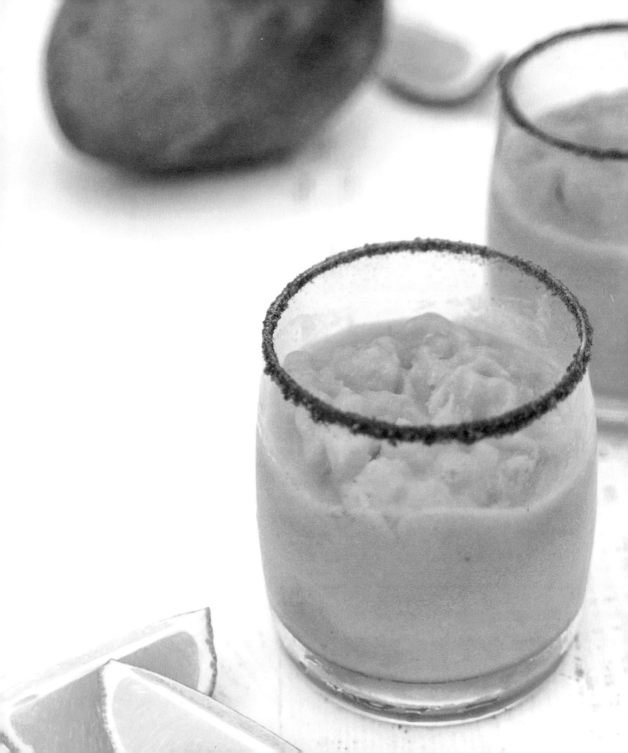

FROZEN MANGO MOCK-A-RITA

SERVES 4

Add a touch of the tropics to the classic Mock-a-rita and you have yourself a match made in paradise. The sweet mango and sour lime deliver both tangy and fruity flavors.

INGREDIENTS

RIM

Chipotle powder or salt

Lime wedges

DRINK

1 cup fresh or frozen mango

2 cups coconut water

½ cup lime juice

½ cup orange juice

4 cups ice

Few shakes salt

Lime wedges for garnish

TOOLS

Blender

PREPARATION

1. Rim four margarita or lowball glasses with chipotle powder or salt (see page 10).

2. Combine all the drink ingredients in a blender and blend until smooth.

3. Divide the blended mixture among the four rimmed glass.

4. Garnish with extra lime.

USE LEFTOVER ORANGE JUICE IN DRESSINGS AND MARINADES. IT PROVIDES NATURAL SWEETNESS AND, OF COURSE, VITAMIN C!

CHOCOLATE HAZELNUT FROZEN-TINI

SERVES 4

Who doesn't love to eat chocolate hazelnut spread by the spoonful? This frozen treat has all the indulgence with zero added sugar.

INGREDIENTS

3 cups hazelnut milk or non-dairy milk of choice

½ cup canned coconut milk

¾ cup hazelnuts

8 pitted Medjool dates

¼ cup cocoa or cacao powder

1 teaspoon vanilla extract

4 cups ice

Dash of salt

Chopped hazelnuts and chocolate shavings for garnish

Non-dairy whipped cream for topping

TOOLS

Blender

PREPARATION

1. Combine all the ingredients in a blender.

2. Blend on high until ingredients are well combined.

3. Divide the mixture among four large glasses, such as pint glasses.

4. Garnish with chopped hazelnuts and chocolate shavings.

SOAKING HAZELNUTS FOR SIX HOURS OR MORE WILL HELP SOFTEN THEM UP AND FACILITATE BLENDING.

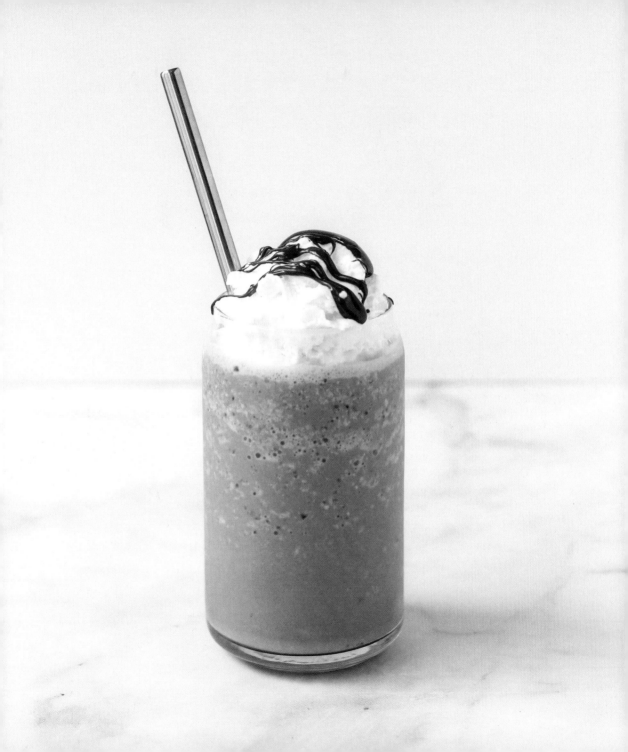

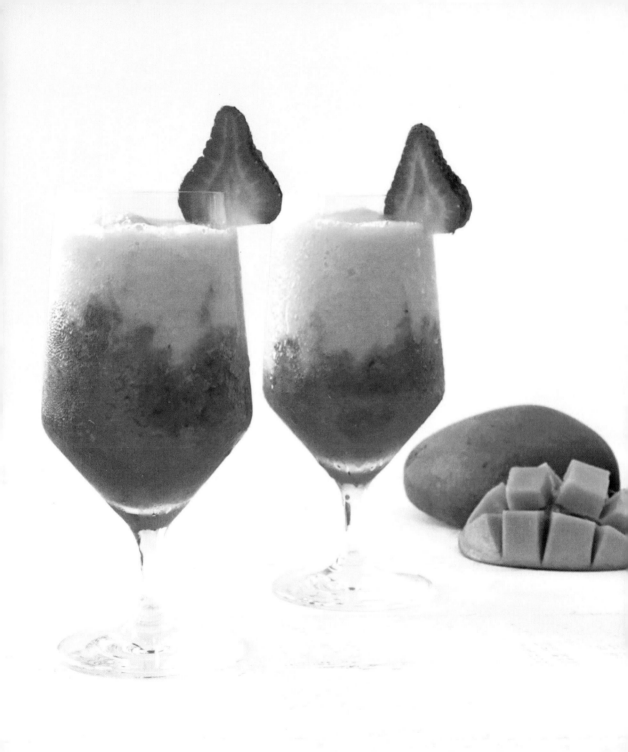

TEQUILA-LESS SUNRISE

You'll get the same beautiful sunrise colors in this frozen, alcohol-free variation
of the classic Tequila Sunrise. Each layer has a unique taste, but the real magic
happens when you mix the two together!

INGREDIENTS

LAYER 1

2 cups frozen mango

1 ½ cups coconut water

2 tablespoons lime juice

1 ½ to 2 cups ice

LAYER 2

2 cups frozen strawberries

1 ½ cups coconut water

2 tablespoons lime juice

4 pitted Medjool dates

1 ½ to 2 cups ice

Lime slices for garnish

TOOLS

Blender

PREPARATION

1. Combine the Layer 1 ingredients in a blender.

2. Blend until smooth, then place in the freezer to keep cold.

3. Meanwhile, combine the Layer 2 ingredients in the blender.

4. Blend on high until the dates are broken up for evenly distributed sweetness.

5. To serve, pour alternating layers of each flavor into four large glasses, such as hurricane glasses, to create a layered effect.

6. Garnish with lime slices.

TALK ABOUT FIBER-RICH! THE MANGO, STRAWBERRIES, AND DATES GIVE THIS DRINK ALMOST 4 GRAMS OF FIBER PER SERVING.

GINGER FROZEN LEMONADE

When life gives you lemons . . . make our zesty and refreshing Ginger Frozen Lemonade! You will never go back to frozen concentrates once you try our lightly sweet and perfectly balanced mocktail.

INGREDIENTS

4 cups coconut water

¾ cup lemon juice

¼ cup agave nectar

¼ cup peeled and chopped fresh ginger

4 cups ice

Twist of lemon for garnish

TOOLS

Blender

PREPARATION

1. Combine all the ingredients in a blender and blend until smooth.

2. Divide the mixture among four highball glasses.

3. Garnish each glass with a twist of lemon.

USE EXTRA GINGER TO MAKE OUR BLACKBERRY MINT MOCKTAIL MULE, FOUND ON PAGE 49.

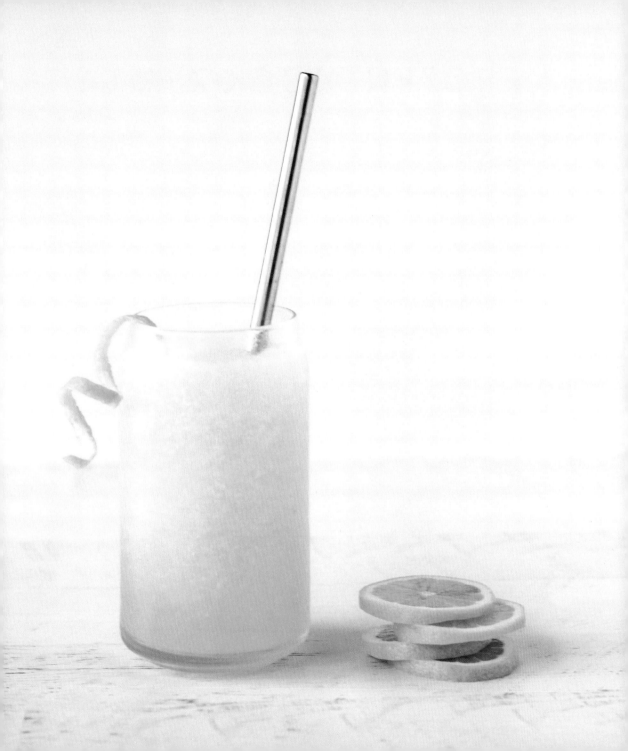

FROZEN MOCK-A-RITA

This frozen variation on our Sour Mock-a-rita is perfect for serving a larger crowd. Throw in extra frozen fruit before blending for natural sweetness—you may not even need the agave!

INGREDIENTS

SALTED RIM

Lime wedges

Sea salt

DRINK

1 cup lime juice, frozen in an ice cube tray at least a few hours in advance or overnight

2 ½ cups coconut water

½ cup orange juice

¼ cup agave nectar

3 cups ice

Lime wedges for garnish

TOOLS

Blender

Ice cube tray

PREPARATION

1. Rim four margarita or lowball glasses with salt (see page 10).

2. Combine all the drink ingredients in a blender and blend until smooth.

3. Divide the blended mixture among the salt-rimmed glasses.

4. Garnish with extra lime.

DO NOT SKIP THE STEP OF FREEZING THE LIME JUICE! THIS IS CRITICAL FOR ACHIEVING A FROZEN, FROTHY MOCKTAIL THAT ISN'T WATERED DOWN BY REGULAR ICE.

FROZEN BAHAMA MAMA

Transport yourself to the tropics with our Frozen Bahama Mama, made with coconut milk and tropical fruit. Bursting with flavor, this drink is a hard one to put down!

INGREDIENTS

2 frozen ripe bananas

1 cup frozen pineapple

1 cup non-dairy milk of choice

1 cup orange juice

1 cup pomegranate juice

½ cup canned coconut milk

2 cups ice

Pineapple and maraschino cherries for garnish

TOOLS

Blender

PREPARATION

1. Combine all the ingredients in a blender.

2. Blend on high until well combined.

3. Divide the mixture among four large glasses, such as hurricane glasses.

4. Garnish with fresh pineapple and maraschino cherries.

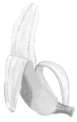

PEEL, SLICE, AND FREEZE RIPE BANANAS FOR LATER USE. REMEMBER, THE RIPER THE BANANA, THE SWEETER THE DRINK!

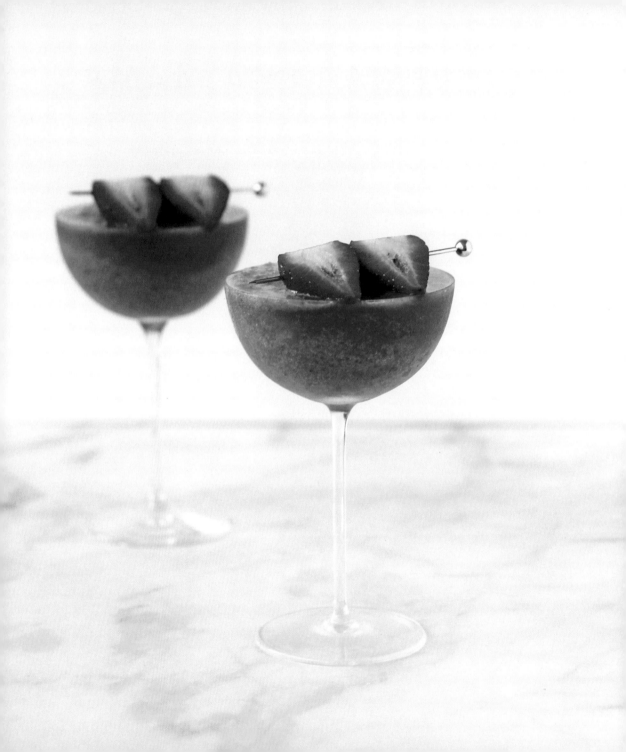

NO WAY FROSÉ

Frosé has become the unofficial drink of summer. Our take on this adult
slushie is both crisp and rich in antioxidants.

INGREDIENTS

2 cups frozen strawberries

1 cup white grape juice

1 cup coconut water

½ cup pomegranate juice (cranberry juice or
tart cherry juice would also be tasty!)

¼ cup lemon juice

2 teaspoons apple cider vinegar

2 cups ice

Fresh strawberries for garnish

TOOLS

Blender

PREPARATION

1. Combine all the ingredients in a blender.

2. Blend on high until well combined.

3. Divide the mixture among four coupes or stemless
   wine glasses.

4. Garnish with extra strawberries.

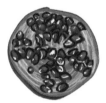

WATERMELON LIME SLUSHIE

What could be more refreshing on a hot summer day than fresh watermelon? How about a frozen watermelon slushie with no added sugar? This is the ultimate poolside mocktail!

INGREDIENTS

5 cups watermelon, cubed and frozen for at least 3 to 4 hours

1 cup coconut water

½ cup lime juice

Few dashes salt

Lime slices for garnish

TOOLS

Blender

PREPARATION

1. Combine all the ingredients in a blender.

2. Blend on high until well combined.

3. Divide the blended mixture among four lowball or margarita glasses.

4. Garnish with lime slices.

TO SERVE IN A MINI WATERMELON AS PICTURED, HOLLOW OUT HALF OF A WATERMELON AND FREEZE THE FRUIT. COVER AND STORE THE WATERMELON RIND IN THE FRIDGE UNTIL READY TO PREPARE YOUR MOCKTAIL. ONE HALF OF A MINI WATERMELON MAKES TWO TO FOUR SERVINGS.

FRESH MINT WOULD BE A DELICIOUS ADDITION TO THIS SLUSHIE!

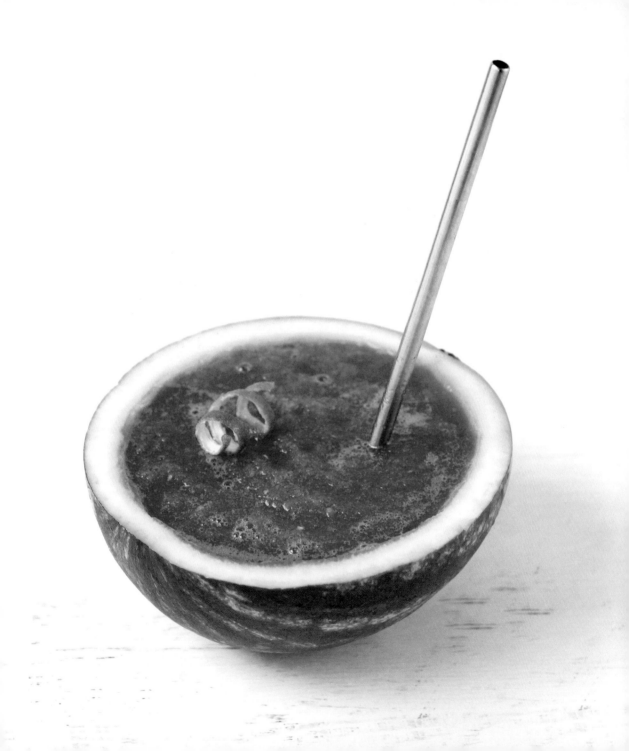

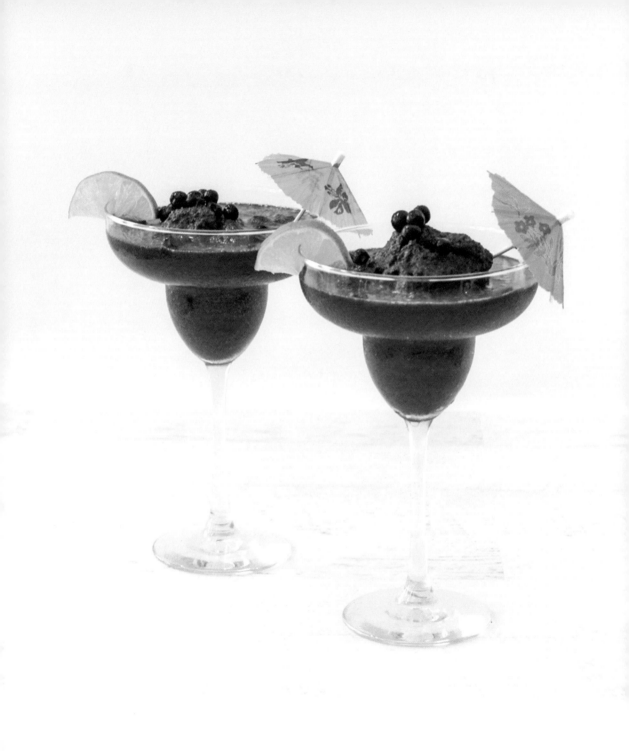

BLUEBERRY AÇAI FROZEN DAIQUIRI

This is not your average, overly sweet virgin Daiquiri. We use açai puree to add richness and body, as well as antioxidants and fiber, to this already nutrient-dense mocktail.

INGREDIENTS

4 frozen unsweetened açai packets (about 3.5 ounces per packet)

2 cups frozen blueberries

1 cup frozen cauliflower or cauliflower rice

8 pitted Medjool dates

4 cups coconut water

¼ cup lime juice

Lime slices for garnish

TOOLS
Blender

PREPARATION

1. Combine all the ingredients in a blender.

2. Blend on high until smooth.

3. Divide the blended mixture among four margarita glasses.

4. Garnish with lime slices.

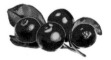

MAKE SURE TO BUY UNSWEETENED AÇAI! WE TESTED THIS RECIPE USING AÇAI FROM SAMBAZON BRAND. AÇAI MAY BE A LITTLE PRICEY, SO FEEL FREE TO USE FEWER PACKS PER SERVING—IT WILL STILL DELIVER ENOUGH FLAVOR AND NUTRITIONAL BENEFITS. IF YOU CAN'T FIND AÇAI OR IT'S NOT YOUR CUP OF TEA, LEAVE IT OUT OR SUBSTITUTE FROZEN FRUIT, SUCH AS RASPBERRIES.

SWEET WINE-NOT SLUSHIE

Frozen grapes are a delicious summer treat. When blended with coconut water, lemon juice, and apple cider vinegar, you get a perfectly sweet, alcohol-free slushie that tastes like it was made with wine!

INGREDIENTS

4 cups frozen green grapes (you can substitute red grapes for a slightly less sweet drink, or swap half of the green grapes with another frozen fruit, like peaches or strawberries)

2 cups coconut water

¼ cup and 2 tablespoons lemon juice

2 teaspoons apple cider vinegar

2 cups ice

Frozen grapes for garnish

TOOLS

Blender

PREPARATION

1. Combine all the ingredients in a blender.

2. Blend on high until the ingredients are well combined.

3. Divide the mixture among four chilled stemless wine glasses.

4. Garnish with extra frozen grapes.

CAN'T FIND FROZEN GRAPES? BUY FRESH ONES AND STORE THEM IN THE FREEZER FOR AT LEAST FOUR HOURS.

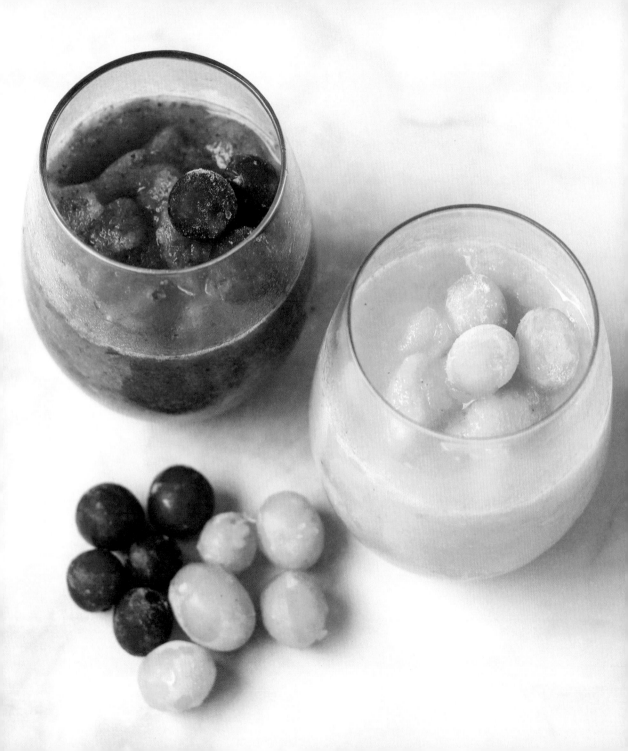

CHAPTER

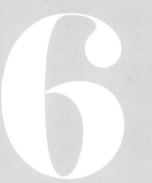

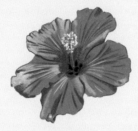

DRINKS WITH BENEFITS

In this section, we crafted mocktails that feature nutrient-dense ingredients, like kombucha, turmeric, and matcha green tea. These ingredients give our drinks vibrant colors and unique flavors in addition to packing a nutritional punch.

WARM LAVENDER BREW

Lavender may help alleviate restlessness, anxiety, and insomnia. This drink will help you wind down after a long day, or keep you calm when you are feeling a little overwhelmed.

INGREDIENTS

2 cups unsweetened non-dairy milk

¼ cup canned coconut milk

2 tablespoons lavender syrup (see page 66)

2 teaspoons vanilla extract

Sprinkle of sea salt

Non-dairy whipped cream for topping

TOOLS

Saucepan

Frother (optional)

PREPARATION

1. Combine all the ingredients in a saucepan over medium heat and bring to a simmer.

2. Simmer on low for 10 minutes (do not allow to boil), whisking periodically to avoid the development of a skin. Alternatively, use a frother to create a foam effect!

3. Divide between two mugs.

4. Top with non-dairy whipped cream.

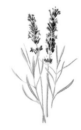

SEE THE SOOTHING SPRITZER RECIPE ON PAGE 66 FOR MORE INFORMATION ON LAVENDER AND HOW TO PREPARE THE LAVENDER SIMPLE SYRUP.

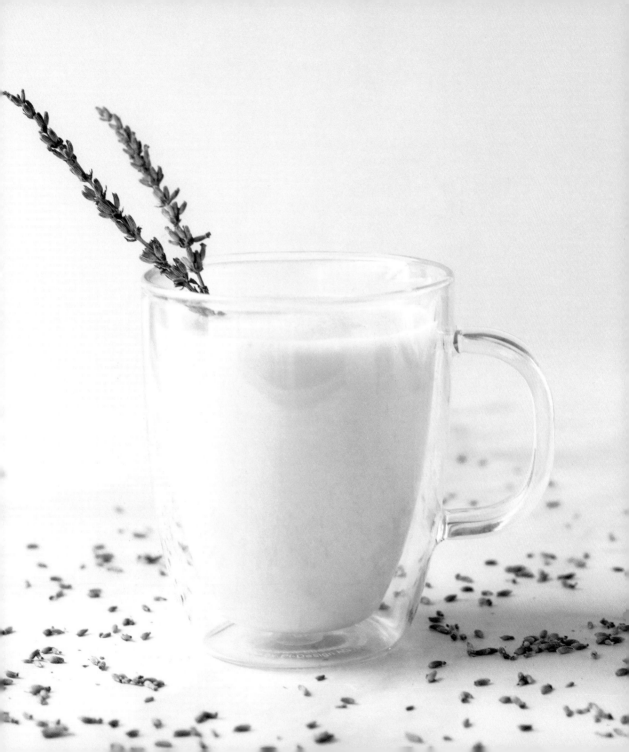

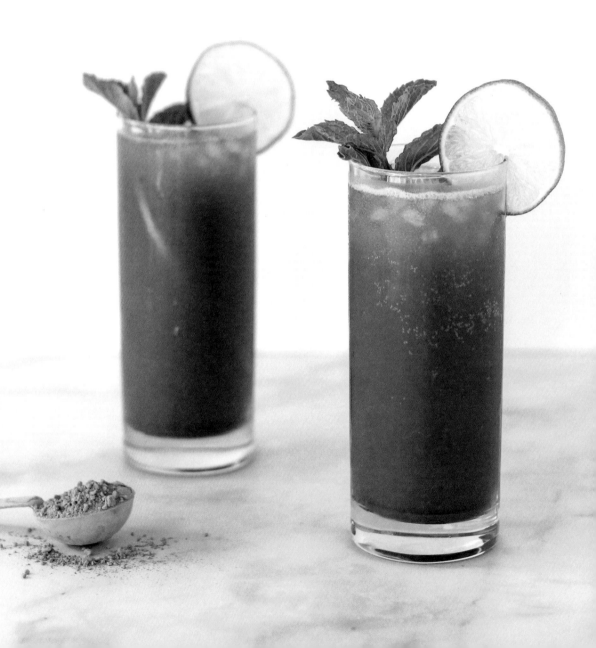

MATCHA MOCK-JITO

Matcha powder is made from finely ground green tea leaves. Like other green teas, matcha contains antioxidants, namely catechins, which have many purported health benefits.

INGREDIENTS

20 mint leaves

1 teaspoon agave nectar

1 cup coconut water

2 tablespoons lime juice

1 teaspoon matcha tea powder

1 cup seltzer

Extra mint sprigs or leaves for garnish

TOOLS

Muddler

Shaker

PREPARATION

1. Muddle the mint leaves with the agave nectar in the bottom of a shaker.

2. Add the coconut water, lime juice, matcha powder, and ice.

3. Shake vigorously.

4. Fill two highball glasses with ice and strain the shaken mixture into the glasses.

5. Top with seltzer (½ cup per serving) and stir.

6. Garnish with mint sprigs.

USE EXTRA MATCHA TO MAKE A MATCHA LATTE: WARM UP MATCHA, COCONUT MILK, AND AGAVE NECTAR FOR A DELICIOUS, SWEET TREAT.

CHIA FRESCA

Citrusy, hydrating, and satisfying, this drink is our take on the chia fresca, which is popular in Latin America. You'll barely notice the chia seeds as you sip but will reap all their amazing benefits, as they are packed with fiber and omega-3 fatty acids.

INGREDIENTS

1 ½ cups coconut or maple water

½ cup grapefruit juice

¼ cup lemon juice

¼ cup orange juice

2 tablespoons chia seeds

½ cup seltzer

Orange, lemon, or grapefruit slices for garnish

PREPARATION

1. Divide all the ingredients except the seltzer between two highball glasses and let sit in the refrigerator for at least 2 hours.

2. When ready to serve, top with seltzer (¼ cup per serving).

3. Garnish with slices of citrus.

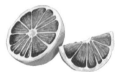

USE EXTRA CHIA SEEDS TO MAKE CHIA SEED PUDDING. COMBINE 2 TABLESPOONS CHIA SEEDS WITH 1/2 CUP NON-DAIRY MILK AND LET SIT IN THE FRIDGE OVERNIGHT. TOP WITH BERRIES.

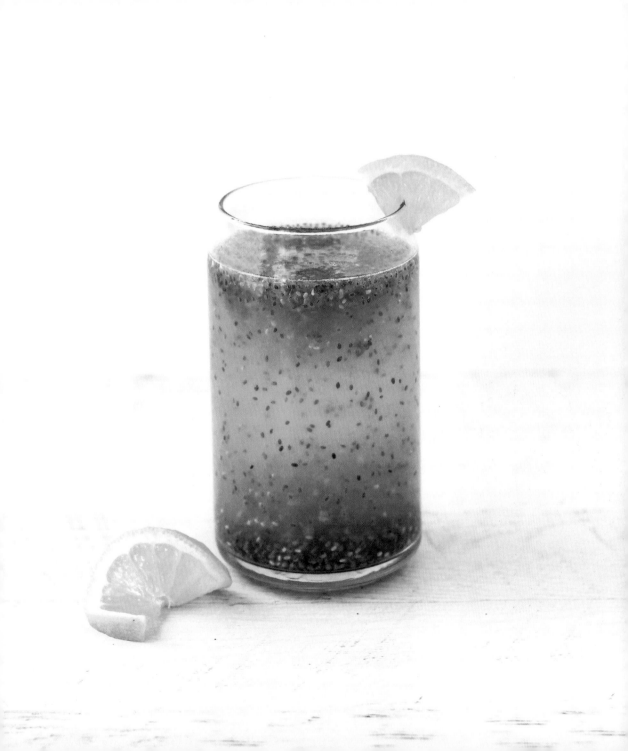

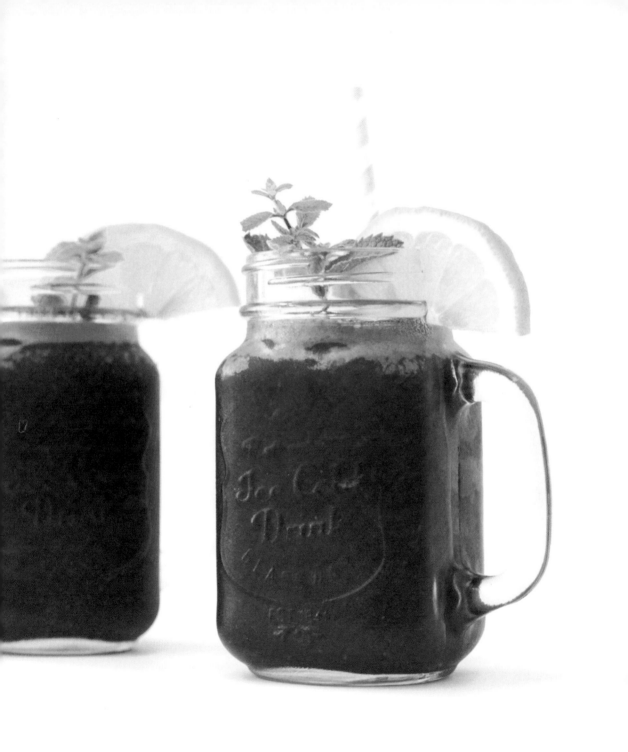

PINK PITAYA LEMONADE

Swap the sugary store-bought pink lemonade for our nutrient-dense version.
It's made with pitaya (also known as dragon fruit) and strawberries, which
provide antioxidants, micronutrients, and fiber.

INGREDIENTS

1 cup frozen pitaya (we made ours with Pitaya brand)

½ cup strawberries, fresh or frozen

2 cups coconut water

½ cup lemon juice

2 tablespoons agave nectar

Lemon slices for garnish

TOOLS

Blender

PREPARATION

1. Combine all the ingredients in a blender and blend until smooth.

2. Divide the blended mixture among highball glasses.

3. Garnish with lemon slices.

CAN'T FIND PITAYA? DOUBLE THE QUANTITY OF STRAWBERRIES OR SWAP
IN YOUR FAVORITE FROZEN FRUIT.

TURMERIC TONIC

Turmeric contains curcumin, which is an antioxidant compound with anti-inflammatory properties. A sprinkle of black pepper helps to facilitate its absorption, which is ordinarily quite poor.

INGREDIENTS

1 ½ cups coconut water

½ cup orange juice

¼ cup lemon juice

2 teaspoons honey or agave nectar

2 teaspoons peeled and chopped fresh ginger

1 teaspoon peeled and chopped fresh turmeric

Couple light shakes of ground black pepper

TOOLS

Blender

Strainer or nut milk bag (optional)

PREPARATION

1. Combine all the ingredients in a blender and blend until smooth.

2. Fill two lowball glasses with ice and divide the mixture between the glasses, or strain into the glasses if desired.

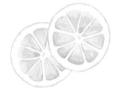

MANGO KALE REFRESHER

If you struggle to reach your veggie intake, this mocktail is for you. The sweetness of the mango masks any taste from the kale, providing a perfect way to get your greens.

INGREDIENTS

2 cups mango, fresh or frozen

1 cup kale

1 cup coconut water

2 tablespoons fresh mint

2 tablespoons lime juice

1 tablespoon agave nectar

Additional mint leaves for garnish

TOOLS

Blender

PREPARATION

1. Combine all the ingredients in a blender.

2. Blend until all ingredients are well combined.

3. Divide the blended mixture between two lowball glasses.

4. Garnish with extra mint leaves.

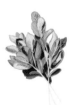

TOSS EXTRA MANGO, KALE, AND MINT TOGETHER TO MAKE A DELICIOUS, REFRESHING SUMMER SALAD.

CHERRY SOUR

Tart cherry juice is touted for its anti-inflammatory benefits. It makes for a unique and colorful take on a Boston Sour.

INGREDIENTS

1 cup maple or coconut water

⅔ cup tart cherry juice

¼ cup lemon juice

1 tablespoon aquafaba

1 tablespoon agave nectar

½ teaspoon apple cider vinegar

Sweet cherries (fresh or frozen) for garnish

TOOLS

Shaker

PREPARATION

1. Combine all the ingredients in a shaker and dry shake (without ice) for 30 seconds.

2. Add ice to the shaker and continue to shake.

3. Strain the shaken mixture into two lowball glasses.

4. Garnish with cherries

SIP ON TART CHERRY JUICE BEFORE OR AFTER INTENSE WORKOUTS TO HELP WITH MUSCLE RECOVERY.

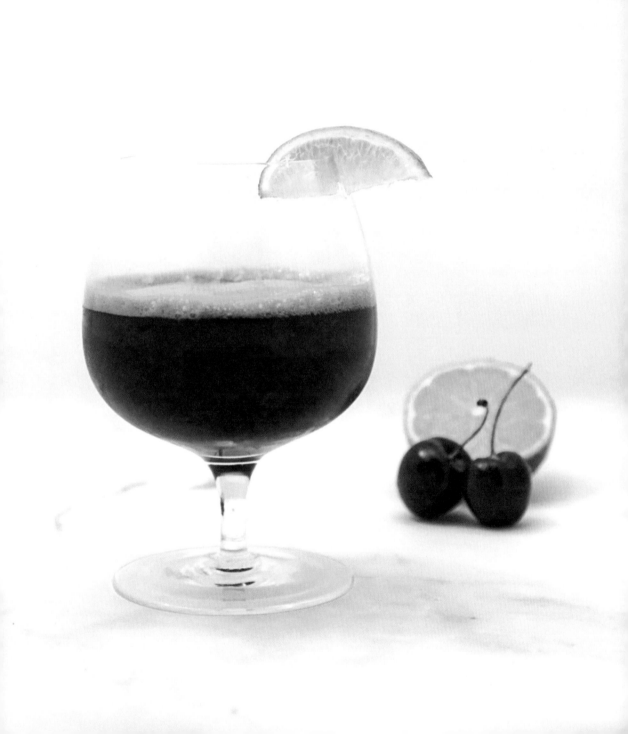

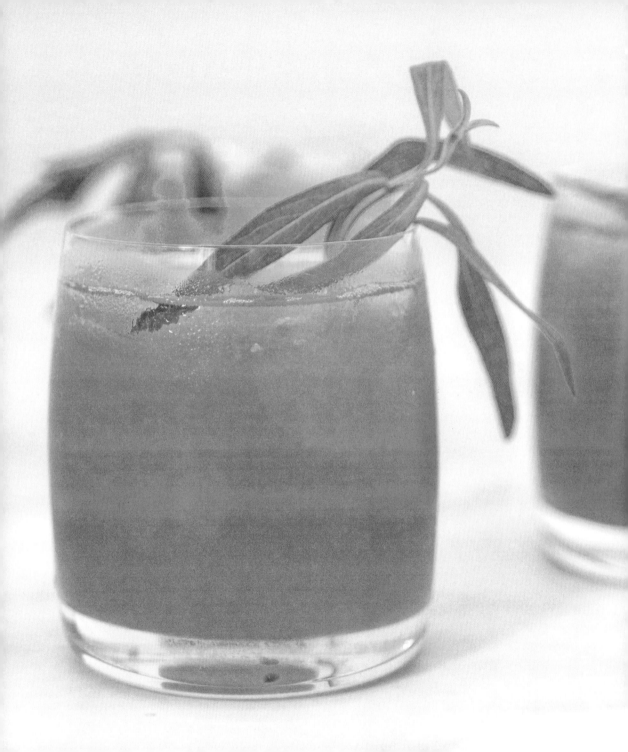

CAROTENE COOLER

This vegetable mocktail tastes bright and fresh and provides you with essential nutrients. Carrots are known for their beta-carotene content—a form of vitamin A. Plus, their natural sweetness lends itself to a delicious beverage with less sugar than fruit juice.

INGREDIENTS

2 large sprigs of fresh tarragon (or ½ teaspoon dried)

2 tablespoons lime juice

1 ½ cups coconut water

¼ cup and 2 tablespoons chopped carrot

¼ cup and 2 tablespoons chopped celery (or cucumber)

1 tablespoon and 1 teaspoon peeled and chopped fresh ginger

Dash of salt

Additional tarragon sprigs for garnish

TOOLS

Blender

Muddler

Shaker

Strainer or nut milk bag

PREPARATION

1. Muddle the tarragon and lime juice in the bottom of a shaker.

2. Combine all the remaining ingredients in a blender and blend until smooth.

3. Strain the blended mixture into the shaker and add ice.

4. Shake vigorously for 30 seconds.

5. Fill two lowball glasses with ice and strain the shaken mixture into the glasses.

6. Garnish with tarragon sprigs.

USE EXTRA CARROTS AND CELERY TO MAKE SOUP, OR PAIR THEM WITH HUMMUS FOR A NUTRITIOUS SNACK.

BLACKBERRY HIBISCUS SPARKLER

SERVES 2

Hibiscus tea, made from hibiscus flowers, is naturally caffeine-free and rich in antioxidants. It adds tartness and a floral element to this bubbly beverage.

INGREDIENTS

⅔ cup blackberries

1 cup brewed hibiscus tea, cooled

2 tablespoons lime juice

1 tablespoon and 1 teaspoon honey

½ teaspoon apple cider vinegar

1 cup seltzer

TOOLS

Muddler

Shaker

Strainer or nut milk bag (optional)

PREPARATION

1. Muddle the blackberries in the bottom of a shaker.

2. Add all the remaining ingredients except the seltzer along with ice.

3. Shake vigorously for 30 seconds.

4. Divide the shaken mixture between highball glasses (option to strain). Top with ice as desired.

5. Top with seltzer (½ cup per serving).

TO STRENGTHEN THE FLAVOR OF THE HIBISCUS TEA, BREW 2 TEA BAGS FOR EVERY 8 OUNCES OF WATER.

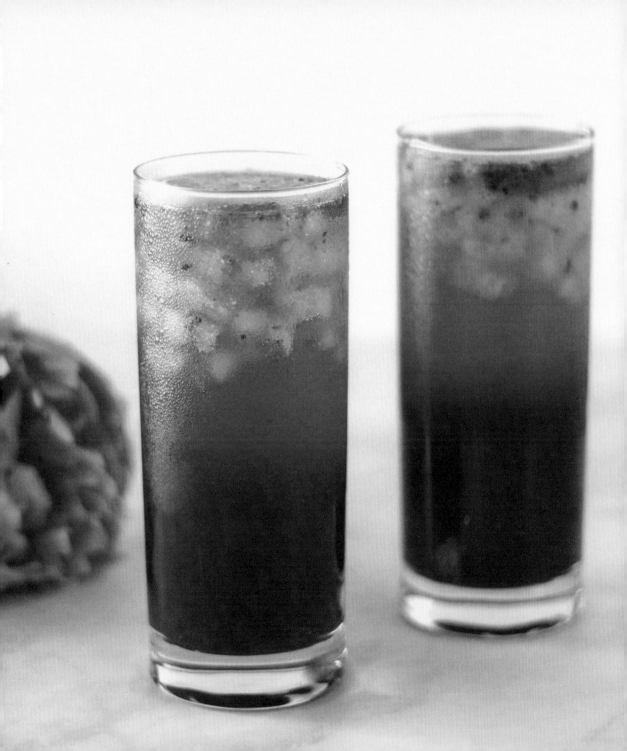

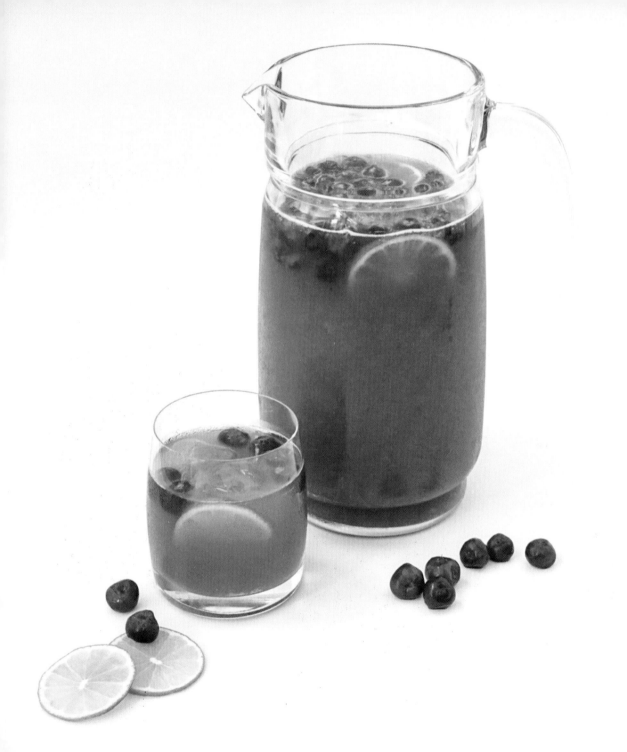

PROBIOTIC PUNCH

Get the party started with our probiotic punch! Kombucha is a fermented tea drink that contains probiotics, an important element of gut health.

INGREDIENTS

3 cups kombucha

2 cups cranberry juice

¾ cup orange juice

¼ cup and 2 tablespoons lime juice

Fresh cranberries and lime wedges for garnish

TOOLS

Pitcher

PREPARATION

1. Combine all the ingredients in a pitcher (this can be prepared ahead of time).

2. To serve, fill six lowball glasses with ice and divide the mixture among the glasses.

3. Garnish with fresh cranberries and lime wedges.

SUGAR IS ESSENTIAL TO THE FERMENTATION PROCESS THAT MAKES KOMBUCHA WHAT IT IS (IT KEEPS THE SCOBY, OR SYMBIOTIC COLONY OF BACTERIA AND YEAST, ALIVE). WITH THAT SAID, LOOK FOR A KOMBUCHA BRAND THAT IS RELATIVELY LOW IN SUGAR (LESS THAN 10 GRAMS PER 8-OUNCE SERVING).

CHAPTER

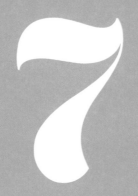

HOLIDAY AND SEASONAL DRINKS

Looking for the perfect drink for a holiday party or special occasion? From New Year's to Valentine's Day to Thanksgiving, we've got you covered. The drinks in this section were designed with specific holidays and seasons in mind, but many of our other mocktail recipes make great additions to parties big and small.

LOVE DRUNK

This mocktail is inspired by the Kir Royale, capturing its sophistication and beautiful hue. Perfect for Valentine's Day or any romantic occasion!

INGREDIENTS

½ cup raspberries

½ cup coconut or maple water

¼ cup grape juice and/or pomegranate juice

½ teaspoon apple cider vinegar

⅔ cup seltzer

Extra raspberries for garnish

TOOLS

Muddler

Shaker

PREPARATION

1. Muddle the raspberries in the bottom of a shaker.

2. Add all the remaining ingredients except the seltzer to the shaker along with ice.

3. Shake vigorously for 30 seconds.

4. Strain the shaken mixture into two champagne glasses.

5. Top with seltzer (⅓ cup per serving).

6. Garnish with raspberries.

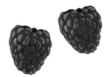

USE EXTRA RASPBERRIES IN SALADS, SMOOTHIES, OR OATMEAL.

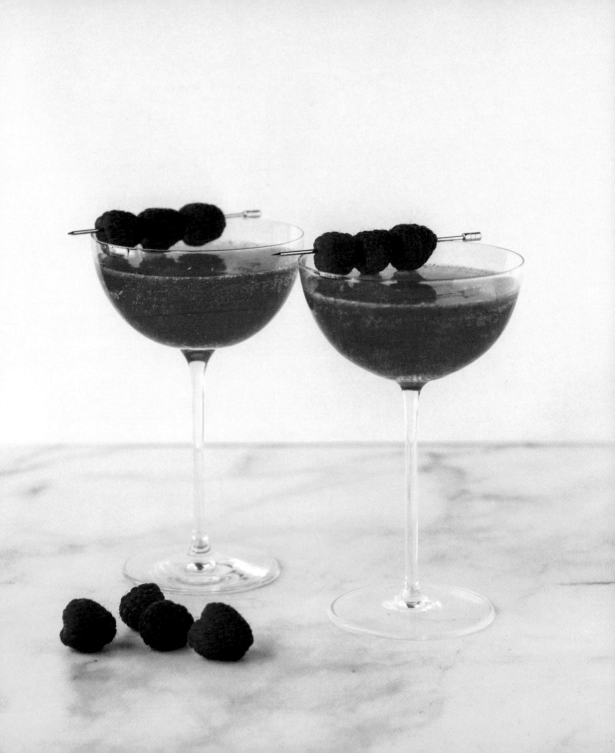

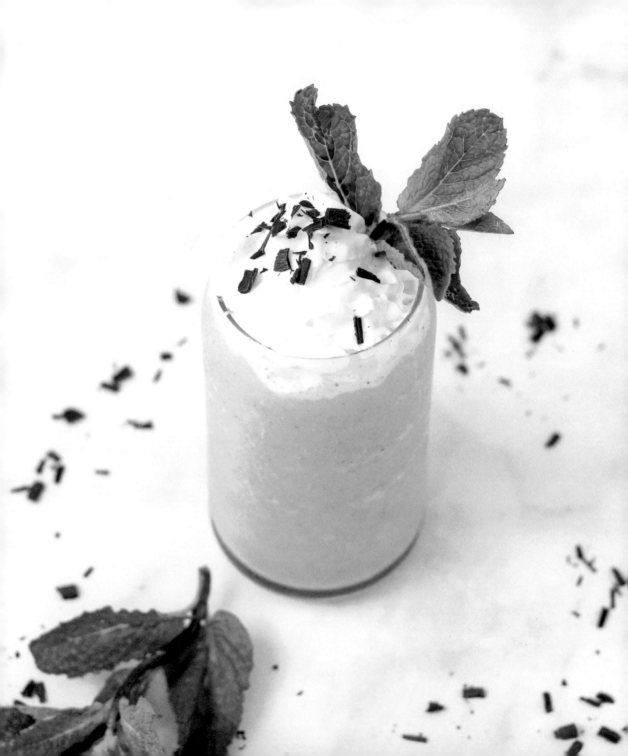

ST. PATRICK'S DAY SHAKE

SERVES 2

Our take on the beloved seasonal green mint shake makes for a festive
St. Patty's Day drink or an anytime delicious green smoothie.

INGREDIENTS

2 ½ cups non-dairy milk

2 frozen bananas

1 cup spinach

½ cup frozen cauliflower or cauliflower rice

¼ teaspoon vanilla extract

¼ teaspoon mint extract, or to taste

1 cup ice

2 tablespoons cacao nibs or chocolate shavings
for garnish

Non-dairy whipped cream for topping

TOOLS

Blender

PREPARATION

1. Combine all the ingredients in a blender. Blend
   until smooth.

2. Divide the mixture between two larger glasses, such as
   pint glasses.

3. Serve topped with whipped cream and cacao nibs or
   chocolate shavings.

DON'T HAVE MINT EXTRACT ON HAND? YOU CAN SUBSTITUTE FRESH
MINT LEAVES (START WITH 4 TO 5 AND INCREASE AS DESIRED FOR A
STRONGER MINT FLAVOR).

FROZEN HURRICANE

Unlike the iconic New Orleans cocktail, our frozen Hurricane will leave you with no regrets. With less juice and no syrups, you'll avoid the sugar hangover that follows most cocktails! A great addition to a Mardi Gras party or a perfect frozen, tropical treat for any ordinary Tuesday.

INGREDIENTS

1 cup passion fruit, fresh or frozen (no sugar added)

1 cup pineapple, fresh or frozen

2 cups pomegranate juice

½ cup orange juice

2 tablespoons lime juice

2 cups ice

Orange slices and maraschino cherries for garnish

TOOLS

Blender

PREPARATION

1. Combine all the ingredients in a blender.

2. Blend on high until smooth and frothy.

3. Divide the blended mixture among four hurricane or other large glasses.

4. Garnish with fresh orange slices and maraschino cherries.

IF POSSIBLE, BUY PASSION FRUIT WITH SEEDS TO REAP THE BENEFITS OF THE ADDED FIBER.

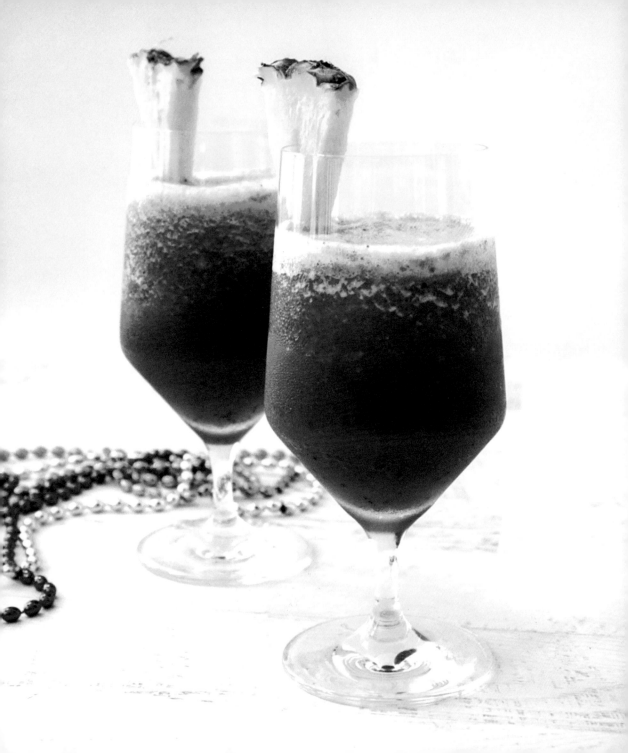

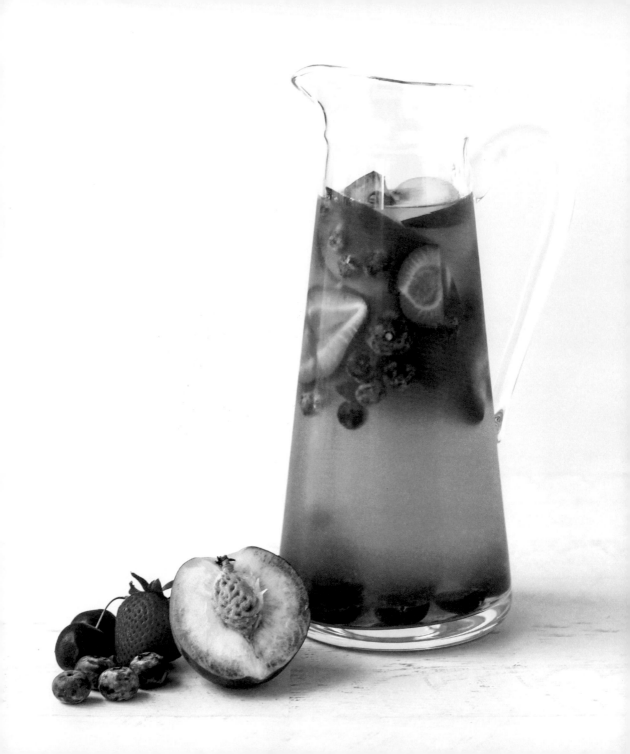

RED, WHITE, AND BLUE SANS-GRIA

What better way to add color to a celebration than with a festive drink?
Perfect for any summer gathering, or 4th of July or Memorial Day party!

INGREDIENTS

2 to 3 cups red, white, and blue fresh fruit (e.g., halved strawberries, blueberries, raspberries, cherries, white peach, or apple sliced or cut into star shapes)

2 ½ cups white grape juice

2 ½ cups coconut water

¼ cup citrus juice (lemon or lime)

1 cup seltzer

Fresh mint for garnish

Additional seltzer for topping

TOOLS

Pitcher

PREPARATION

1. Place the sliced fruit in a large pitcher.

2. Add the white grape juice, coconut water, and citrus juice and stir well.

3. Place in the refrigerator and let chill for 3 to 4 hours.

4. When ready to serve, top with the seltzer and stir.

5. Fill six lowball or stemless wine glasses with ice. Divide the mixture, including the fruit, among the glasses.

6. Garnish with fresh mint and top with additional seltzer.

PUMPKIN SPICE LATTE

Pumpkin Spice Lattes have become the official drink of fall. Make your own lower-sugar version at home, no espresso machine required!

INGREDIENTS

2 cups non-dairy milk

1 ½ cups strong brewed coffee

¼ cup canned coconut milk

1 tablespoon and 1 teaspoon agave nectar

½ teaspoon vanilla extract

2 teaspoons pumpkin pie spice

Additional pumpkin pie spice for garnish

TOOLS

Saucepan

Frother (optional)

Shaker

PREPARATION

HOT VERSION

1. Combine all the ingredients in a saucepan over medium heat, and slowly bring to a simmer as you stir.

2. Whisk until the mixture is well combined. Option to use a frother.

3. Divide the drink between two large (16-ounce) mugs. Top with a dash of pumpkin pie spice.

ICED VERSION

1. Allow the coffee to completely cool, or use cold brew coffee.

2. Combine all the ingredients in a shaker and add ice.

3. Shake vigorously for 30 seconds.

4. Fill two pint glasses with ice and strain the shaken mixture into the glasses.

ADD UP TO 2 TABLESPOONS OF PUMPKIN PUREE (OR 1 TABLESPOON PER SERVING) TO THE MIXTURE WHILE WHISKING FOR A BOOST OF VITAMIN A. IT'S A GREAT WAY TO USE UP EXTRA PUMPKIN!

MULLED WINE-NOT

This mulled mocktail recipe is cozy, spicy, and the perfect accompaniment to a winter gathering or a night by the fire.

INGREDIENTS

3 cups pomegranate juice or grape juice (no sugar added)

3 cups coconut water

½ cup orange juice

Zest of ½ orange

Zest of ½ lemon

12 whole cloves

4 cinnamon sticks

¼ teaspoon ground nutmeg

¼ teaspoon ground cardamom

Lemon and orange slices and cinnamon sticks for garnish

TOOLS

Saucepan

Strainer or nut milk bag

PREPARATION

1. Combine all the ingredients in a saucepan over medium heat. Bring to a simmer.

2. Reduce heat to medium-low. Stir frequently for 15 minutes.

3. Strain the mixture into six mugs.

4. Garnish with fresh lemon slices, orange slices, and cinnamon sticks.

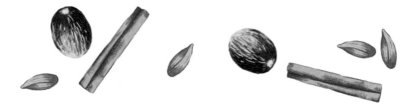

WARM CIDER AND SAGE

This earthy and spicy mocktail is a unique spin on hot cider and will keep you warm on a crisp fall day.

INGREDIENTS

2 ⅔ cups 100% apple juice

2 ⅔ cups maple or coconut water

1 tablespoon and 1 teaspoon apple cider vinegar

12 sage leaves

Few shakes pumpkin pie spice

Additional pumpkin pie spice and sage leaves for garnish

TOOLS

Saucepan

Strainer or nut milk bag (optional)

PREPARATION

1. Combine all the ingredients in a saucepan over medium heat, and slowly bring to a simmer as you stir.

2. Simmer for 3 to 5 minutes to allow the flavors of the sage to steep.

3. Divide the mixture among four mugs (option to strain the sage leaves).

4. Garnish with a dash of pumpkin pie spice and sage leaves.

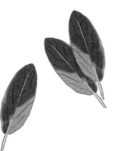

USE EXTRA SAGE TO MAKE OUR APEROL-LESS SPRITZ OR HONEY SAGE SOUR RECIPES, ON PAGES 23 AND 46, RESPECTIVELY.

THIS DRINK IS ALSO DELICIOUS WHEN SHAKEN WITH ICE AND SERVED CHILLED.

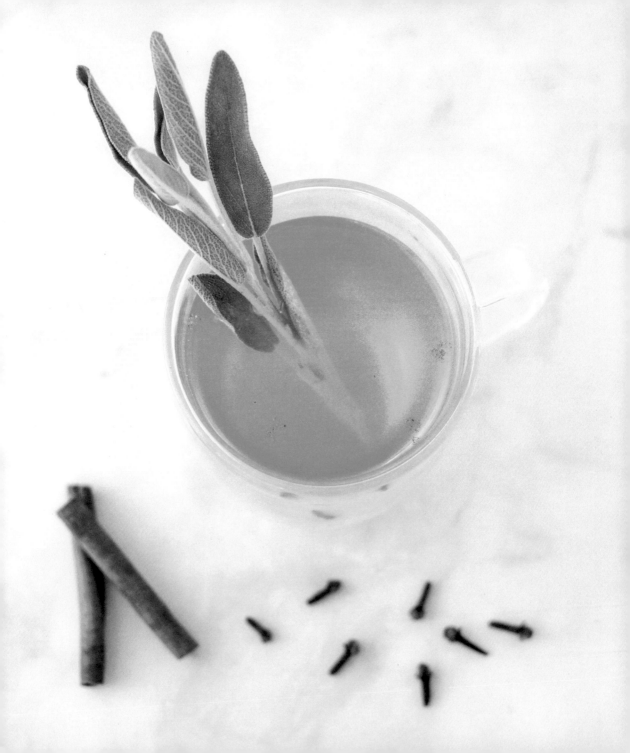

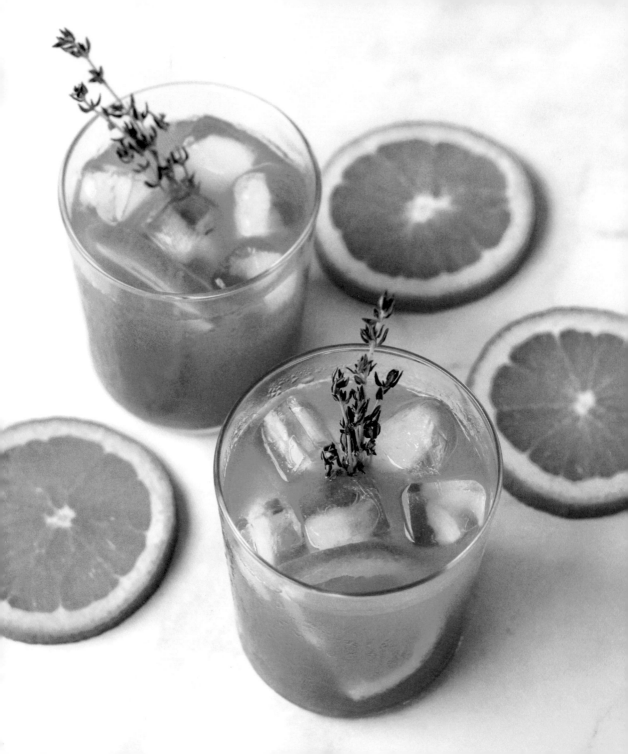

FESTIVE FIZZ

SERVES 2

Made with cranberry juice and fresh thyme, this mocktail is the perfect accompaniment to Thanksgiving dinner, but it's equally fantastic at any time of the year!

INGREDIENTS

4 sprigs fresh thyme

2 teaspoons peeled and chopped fresh ginger

⅔ cup cranberry juice

¼ cup and 2 tablespoons orange juice

1 cup seltzer

Additional thyme and fresh cranberries for garnish

TOOLS

Muddler

Shaker

PREPARATION

1. Muddle the thyme and ginger in the bottom of a shaker.

2. Add the cranberry and orange juices and fill the shaker with ice. Shake vigorously.

3. Fill two lowball glasses with ice and strain the shaken mixture into the glasses.

4. Top with seltzer (½ cup per serving) and stir.

5. Garnish with thyme sprigs and fresh cranberries.

PEPPERMINT HOT CHOCOLATE

SERVES 4

Swap the peppermint schnapps for peppermint extract to give this hot chocolate a booze-free holiday kick. This soothing, velvety drink will be your new go-to for snowy winter days!

INGREDIENTS

4 cups non-dairy milk

½ cup canned coconut milk

¼ cup maple syrup or agave nectar

1 teaspoon vanilla

½ teaspoon mint extract

2 tablespoons unsweetened cocoa powder or cacao powder

2 ounces dark chocolate

Crushed peppermint candy cane for garnish

Non-dairy whipped cream for topping

TOOLS

Saucepan

PREPARATION

1. Combine all the ingredients in a saucepan over medium heat, and slowly bring to a simmer as you stir. Do not allow the mixture to boil.

2. Whisk until the mixture is well combined.

3. Taste the hot chocolate and add more sweetener if desired for a sweeter drink.

4. Divide among four mugs.

5. Garnish with whipped cream and crushed peppermint candy.

ADD A MINT SPRIG TO THE SIMMERING MIXTURE FOR AN EXTRA BURST OF MINT FLAVOR. IF YOU SERVE WITH A CANDY CANE, IT WILL MELT AND ADD ADDITIONAL PEPPERMINT FLAVOR!

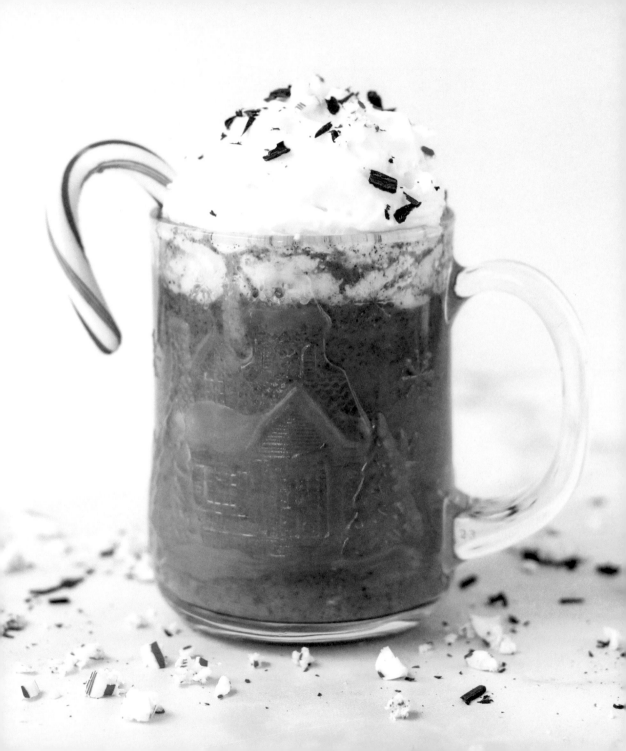

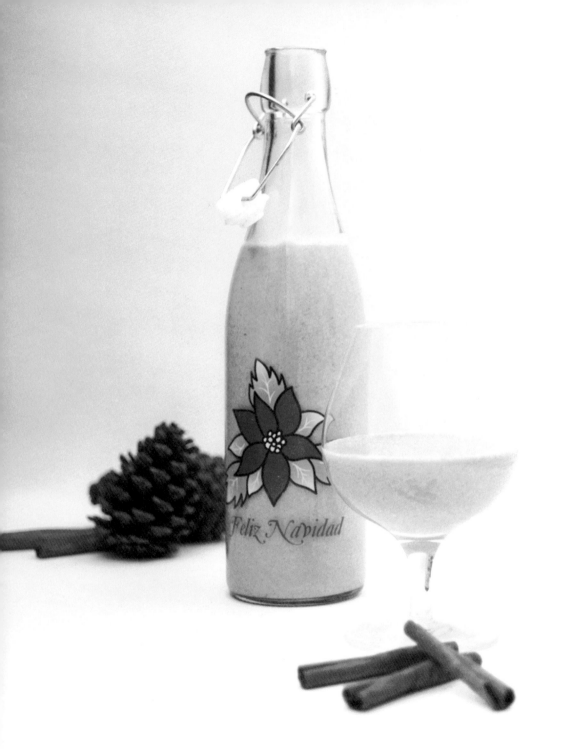

COQUITO

Coquito, also known as Puerto Rican eggnog, is traditionally made with condensed milk and sugar. We adapted this classic Christmas beverage to create a lighter, naturally sweet, plant-based treat without sacrificing any of the flavor.

INGREDIENTS

1 cup raw cashews

8 pitted Medjool dates

3 cups non-dairy milk

¾ cup canned coconut milk

2 teaspoons vanilla extract

2 teaspoons ground cinnamon

1 teaspoon ground nutmeg

1 teaspoon rum extract (optional)

Additional ground cinnamon for garnish

TOOLS

Blender

Pitcher

Strainer or nut milk bag

PREPARATION

1. Soak the cashews and dates in water for at least 6 hours or overnight (the longer you soak, the easier it will be to blend).

2. Drain, then place the cashews and dates in a blender.

3. Add all the remaining ingredients to the blender and blend until smooth.

4. Strain the mixture into a pitcher.

5. Cool the mixture in the fridge for 3 to 4 hours.

6. Serve in lowball glasses with a dash of cinnamon.

ALTHOUGH IT'S TYPICALLY SERVED COLD, YOU CAN ALSO HEAT UP THIS BEVERAGE FOR A DELICIOUS WARM CONCOCTION.

HOLIDAY SPRITZER

SERVES 2

This effervescent mocktail looks and tastes festive and would be perfect for sipping with Christmas breakfast or for toasting with on New Year's Eve. What better way to kick off your resolutions than to make a non-alcoholic drink with antioxidant-rich pomegranate juice?

INGREDIENTS

1 sprig rosemary

⅔ cup 100% pomegranate juice

2 teaspoons lime juice

½ teaspoon apple cider vinegar

1 to 1 ½ cups seltzer

Additional rosemary and pomegranate arils for garnish

TOOLS

Muddler

Shaker

PREPARATION

1. Muddle the rosemary in the bottom of a shaker.

2. Add the pomegranate juice, lime juice, apple cider vinegar, and ice.

3. Shake vigorously for 30 seconds.

4. Strain the mixture into two champagne flutes.

5. Top with seltzer (½ - ¾ cup per serving) and stir.

6. Garnish with rosemary and pomegranate arils.

MAKE SURE TO BUY 100% POMEGRANATE JUICE, NOT CONCENTRATES OR COCKTAILS.

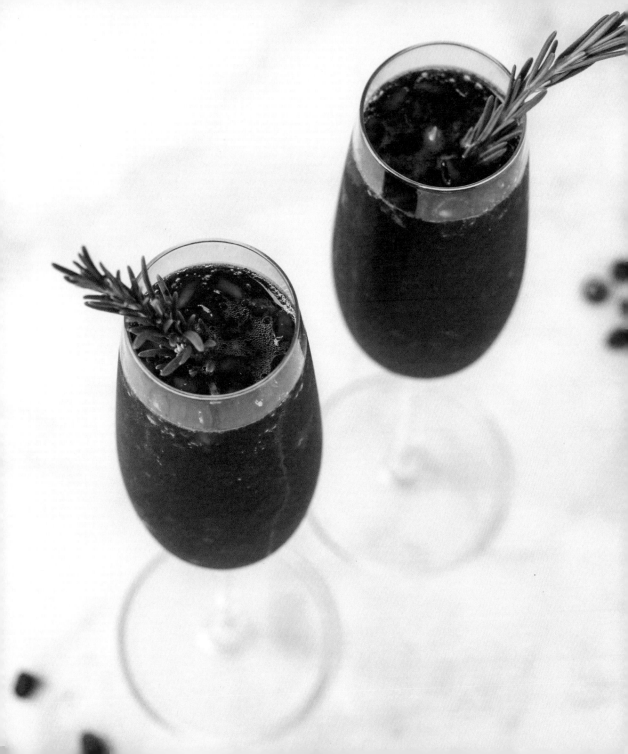

APPENDIX 1:
ALCOHOL STATISTICS AND TRENDS

In this section, we provide more detailed information on alcohol use and abuse. Alcohol use is prevalent in the U.S. The 2018 National Survey on Drug Use and Health (NSDUH) revealed that the majority of U.S. adults—70%—drank in the past year, with 55% reporting that they consumed alcohol within the past month. Among those who participated in the survey, 26% engaged in binge drinking, and 7% reported partaking in heavy alcohol use, defined as five or more binge drinking episodes within the past month. A recent study revealed that high-risk drinking behaviors increased by 30% between 2001 and 2013. In women specifically, this number rose by 58%. Unfortunately, alcohol use disorder affects over 14 million Americans and appears to be on the rise both in the U.S. and globally.

Alcohol consumption is a leading preventable cause of death in the U.S. and globally. A study conducted by the Centers for Disease Control (CDC) found that 88,000 deaths a year can be attributed to alcohol consumption. Furthermore, in 2016, alcohol was found to be a leading cause of death for people age 15-49 years old. Short-term consequences of excessive alcohol intake include alcohol poisoning, harm to a developing fetus during pregnancy, and impaired judgment, which can lead to injury, violence, and risky sexual behaviors. In the long term, excessive alcohol consumption increases the risk of alcoholism, mental health disorders, and chronic diseases, including heart disease, liver disease, and several types of cancer.

With that said, emerging evidence suggests that drinking trends may be changing. Younger generations, namely Generation Z, are imbibing less than previous ones when they were the same age. When asked about the reasons for this shift, Gen Zers cited health concerns, costs associated with "going out," and diminished appeal. In addition, movements like "Dry January" and "Sober October," which invite people to take a month-long break from alcohol, are growing in popularity. This shift toward alcohol-free alternatives has caused a spike in non-alcoholic beer sales. Mocktail bars are also popping up across the U.S., and companies are racing to develop zero-proof spirits.

GETTING HELP
If you are concerned about your or a loved one's alcohol use, talk openly with a healthcare provider. The NIAAA offers reliable online resources (www.niaaa. nih.gov/alcohol-health/support-treatment), including a Treatment Navigator, which contains information about how to talk with a medical provider, evidence-based treatment options, and cost and insurance coverage. The Substance Abuse and Mental Health Services Administration (SAMHSA) maintains a free and confidential hotline at 1-800-662-HELP (4357) and provides information and treatment referrals in English and Spanish 24/7, 365 days a year. You can find additional information and resources on their website at www.findtreatment.gov.

APPENDIX 2:

NOTES FOR WOMEN WHO ARE PREGNANT

Most of the drinks in *Mocktail Party* are safe for pregnant women to consume, with a few exceptions. Here, we provide some information and guidance on making mocktails for women who are pregnant or trying to conceive. As a reminder, our first mocktail book, *Drinking for Two: Nutritious Mocktails for the Mom-to-Be*, was specifically designed with pregnant women in mind and makes a great gift for moms or moms-to-be!

FOOD SAFETY

Food safety is important, particularly during pregnancy. Here are some food safety tips related to making mocktails:

1. Always wash hands prior to and after handling food. Sanitize kitchen surfaces and keep your fridge clean. Use separate cutting boards for raw meat, fish, and produce.
2. Wash your produce with clean water—do not use soaps or detergents. Cut off bruises and other damaged spots.
3. Avoid unpasteurized juices, including freshly squeezed juices purchased at farmers' markets, restaurants, and juice bars.

INGREDIENTS TO USE WITH CAUTION

Açai: We could not find any concrete evidence regarding the consumption of açai during pregnancy. Therefore, we recommend caution if you choose to make our Blueberry Açai Daiquiri. We do not recommend consumption of açai in a powder or supplemental form.

Caffeine: A handful of our drinks are made with tea and coffee, which contain caffeine. The current recommendation for pregnant women is to limit the intake of caffeine to less than 200 milligrams per day. This translates to roughly one-and-a-half cups of coffee a day, depending on the brew; teas typically have less caffeine. Depending on how much caffeine you want to consume during your pregnancy, feel free to use decaf brews or avoid these drinks altogether.

Extracts: Vanilla and other extracts are typically prepared in alcohol (see Extracts section for more information). Consider purchasing or making a non-alcoholic version of these extracts. You can also use ingredients like vanilla bean or fresh mint to flavor drinks.

Herbal Teas: Use caution when consuming herbal teas. The safety of many herbs has not been well-studied in pregnant women, and some teas contain ingredients that may not be safe for consumption during pregnancy. We recommend modifying or avoiding the Blackberry Hibiscus Sparkler, made with hibiscus tea, as well as the drinks made with lavender.

Kombucha: Kombucha is touted for its probiotic content and potential gut-health benefits. However, it is unpasteurized and typically contains at least trace amounts of alcohol. If kombucha is prepared or stored improperly, the fermentation process can continue and produce more alcohol. Some kombuchas are specifically brewed to be alcoholic beverages. There is no known safe amount of alcohol to consume during pregnancy. Out of an abundance of caution and due to uncertainty regarding alcohol content of kombucha, we chose not to include kombucha in our recipes for *Drinking for Two*, and we recommend avoiding or modifying our Mocktail Mule and Probiotic Punch recipes.

Sugar Substitutes: Most sugar substitutes are designated by the FDA as Generally Recognized as Safe (GRAS) for consumption during pregnancy. There is limited scientific evidence available on monk fruit sweetener use during pregnancy. Erythritol, a sugar alcohol, is an additive in some brands of monk fruit sweetener. Limited evidence does not suggest any adverse outcomes associated with moderate erythritol consumption during pregnancy.

APPENDIX 3:

TIPS FOR ADOPTING AN ALCOHOL-FREE LIFESTYLE

Whether it is for a week, a month, or forever, giving up alcohol can have its challenges. Here are some tips to make the transition easier:

• Focus on what you are gaining, not what you are giving up.

• If you know you'll be at a social gathering where alcohol will be present, bring your own alcohol-free alternatives or think about what you'll order instead. Look up menus ahead of time. (Check out our tips for ordering healthy mocktails at a restaurant or bar.)

• Plan how you will respond to people who may ask why you aren't drinking (not that it's anyone's business!) or who may try to derail you. For example, if you are going out with a group, you can offer to be the designated driver.

• Have an alternative in hand. We've found that no one really notices that you aren't imbibing if you are sipping on something. Plus, you won't feel like you are missing out.

• Have fun taste testing all the new non-alcoholic brands popping up!

• Serve mocktails in proper glassware (i.e. in a wine glass or lowball glass). We find that this adds to the experience.

• Observe how you feel when you don't drink. Do you notice any positive changes to your sleeping habits? Anxiety? Skin? Enjoy the feeling of not being hungover!

• Find alternative methods for practicing self-care and coping with stress, such as journaling, calling a friend, going for a walk, taking a bath, or doing yoga.

• Don't go at it alone. Find support from family, friends, or social media groups. Share your delicious mocktail and alcohol-free recipes.

• Use an app to track your alcohol-free days. This helps keep you accountable and motivated.

• When things get tough, remind yourself of why you're doing it in the first place. Remember, taking a break from alcohol can improve your health and save you a lot of money!

• Reward yourself when you reach certain milestones. Reached 30 days without drinking? Treat yourself with a trip to the spa!

TIPS FOR ORDERING MOCKTAILS AT A RESTAURANT OR BAR

• **Avoid sodas and tonic water.** Choose unsweetened seltzer instead.

• **Avoid drink mixes** (such as Margarita mix) and creamy, frozen, and "-ade" drinks. These are calorie and sugar bombs!

• **Add a splash of juice to seltzer or water for flavor.** Or, cut juice with an equal amount of seltzer water to decrease the sugar content. While all juices have something to offer in the way of nutrients, pomegranate and cranberry juice are particularly high in antioxidants. Be sure to avoid juice cocktails and nectars.

• **Choose unsweetened teas over sweetened.** Add sweetener to taste.

• Infuse flavor into drinks by asking for herbs, spices (like cinnamon), or pieces of fresh fruit, like lemon, lime, or orange.

• **Ask the bartender to transform your favorite traditional drinks into alcohol-free and low-sugar versions.** Mojitos, Margaritas (on the rocks), and Bloody Marys, to name a few, can be easily made without the addition of alcohol. Instead of sugar, ask for your drink to be made with a small amount of flavored or infused simple syrup (less than ½ fluid ounce or 1 tablespoon). A little can go a long way, especially for strong flavors, like ginger.

APPENDIX 4:
SUSTAINABLE MIXOLOGY

In line with our plant-based lifestyles, we aim to be sustainable while cooking and mixing up mocktails. Here are a few suggestions for keeping waste to a minimum:

AT THE STORE
• Use eco-friendly produce bags and tote bags for groceries.

• Choose glass containers over plastic containers when possible; for example, look for premade juices in glass bottles.

• Visit your local farmers' market or look for local and seasonal ingredients at the store.

IN THE KITCHEN
• Freeze unused produce before it spoils—or buy frozen produce to begin with.

• Compost leftover produce.

• Zest citrus fruits before juicing. Zest can be used to add flavor to drinks, baked goods, salad dressings, and even savory dishes.

• Use leftover canned coconut milk in Indian or Asian dishes, or to make your own vegan ice cream!

• Grow your own herbs at home.

• Freeze extra herbs for later: Simply chop the herbs and freeze with water in ice cube trays. Add to your sauté pan when cooking, and the water will evaporate.

• Coordinate your drink recipes with food recipes to reduce the risk of throwing away unused herbs. We provide suggestions throughout the book!

BIBLIOGRAPHY

WHY MOVE TO MOCKTAILS?

ALCOHOL AND HEALTH

Terminology Table (Page 2):
"Alcohol Use and Your Health." Centers for Disease Control and Prevention. Last reviewed December 30, 2019. Retrieved from: https://www.cdc.gov/alcohol/fact-sheets/alcohol-use.htm

"Drinking Levels Defined." National Institute on Alcohol Abuse and Alcoholism. Retrieved from: https://www.niaaa.nih.gov/alcohol-health/overview-alcohol-consumption/moderate-binge-drinking

"The American Heart Association..." (Page 3):
"Is drinking alcohol part of a healthy lifestyle?" American Heart Association. Last reviewed December 30, 2019. Retrieved from: https://www.heart.org/en/healthy-living/healthy-eating/eat-smart/nutrition-basics/alcohol-and-heart-health

"...American Cancer Society..." (Page 3):
"Alcohol Use and Cancer." American Cancer Society. Last reviewed June 9, 2020. Retrieved from: https://www.cancer.org/cancer/cancer-causes/diet-physical-activity/alcohol-use-and-cancer.html

"...2020-2025 Dietary Guidelines for Americans..." (Page 3):
U.S. Department of Agriculture and U.S. Department of Health and Human Services. Dietary Guidelines for Americans, 2020-2025.
9th Edition. December 2020. Available at http://www.dietaryguidelines.gov/

"...one drink per day for both men and women." (Page 3):
"Scientific Report of the 2020 Dietary Guidelines Advisory Committee." U.S. Department of Health and Human Services and U.S. Department of Agriculture. First print: July 2020. Retrieved from: https://www.dietaryguidelines.gov/sites/default/files/2020-07/ScientificReport_of_the_2020DietaryGuidelinesAdvisoryCommittee_first-print.pdf

"...one drink per day as well." (Page 3):
Corliss, J. "Is red wine actually good for your health?". Harvard Health Publishing, Harvard School of Medicine. Last updated January 29, 2020. Retrieved from: https://www.health.harvard.edu/blog/is-red-wine-good-actually-for-your-heart-2018021913285

"...with decreased risk of Type 2 Diabetes..." (Page 3):
Xiao-Hua, L., Fei-fei Y., Yu-Hao, Z., Jia, H. "Association between alcohol consumption and the risk of incident type 2 diabetes: a systematic review and dose-response meta-analysis." The American Journal of Clinical Nutrition, Volume 103, Issue 3, Published March 2016. Pages 818–829. Retrieved from: https://doi.org/10.3945/ajcn.115.114389

"...and cardiovascular disease." (Page 3):
Ronksley, Paul E., Brien, Susan E. Turner, Barbara J., Mukamal, Kenneth J., Ghali, William A. "Association of alcohol consumption with selected cardiovascular disease outcomes: a systematic review and meta-analysis." 2011;342:d671. Published February 22, 2011. Retrieved from: hhtps://doi.org/10.1136/bmj.d671

"...various markers of cardiovascular health" (Page 3):
Haseeb, S., Alexander, B., Baranchuk, A. "Wine and Cardiovascular Health: A Comprehensive Review." Circulation. 106(15)1434-1448. Published October 10, 2017. Retrieved from: https://www.ahajournals.org/doi/10.1161/CIRCULATIONAHA.117.030387

"...such as esophageal cancer." **(Page 3):**
"Alcohol and Cancer Risk." National Cancer Institute. Last reviewed September 13, 2018. Retrieved from: https://www.cancer.gov/about-cancer/causes-prevention/risk/alcohol/alcohol-fact-sheet

"...increased risk of breast cancer." **(Page 3):**
Cao, Y., Willett, W., Rimm, E., Stampfer, M., Giovannucci, E. "Light to moderate intake of alcohol, drinking patterns, and risk of cancer: results from two prospective US cohort studies." BMJ. 351, h4238. Published August 18, 2015. Retrieved from: http://doi.org/10.1136/bmj.h4238

"...increased risk of mortality." **(Page 3):**
Wood, A., Kapotge, S., Butterworth, A., Willeit, P., Warnakula, S., Bolton, T., et al. "Risk thresholds for alcohol consumption: combined analysis of individual-participant data for 599 912 current drinkers in 83 prospective studies". The Lancet, Volume 391, Issue 10129, 1513 - 1523. Published April 14, 2018. Retrieved from: https://doi.org/10.1016/S0140-6736(18)30134-X

"...results are nevertheless compelling." **(Page 4):**
Mehta, G., Macdonald, S., Cronberg, A., et al. "Short-term abstinence from alcohol and changes in cardiovascular risk factors, liver function tests and cancer-related growth factors: a prospective observational study." BMJ Open, 8:e020673. First published May 5, 2018. Retrieved from: https://doi.org/10.1136/bmjopen-2017-020673

ADDED SUGARS

"...2020-2025 Dietary Guidelines for Americans ..." **(Page 5):**
"2020-2025 Dietary Guidelines for Americans." U.S. Department of Agriculture and U.S. Department of Health and Human Services. Dietary Guidelines for Americans, 2020-2025. 9th Edition. December 2020. Available at http://www.dietaryguidelines.gov/

"...9 teaspoons for men." **(Page 5):**
"Added Sugars." American Heart Association. Last Reviewed April 17, 2018. Retrieved from: https://www.heart.org/en/healthy-living/healthy-eating/eat-smart/sugar/added-sugars

SUGAR SUBSTITUTES

"...negatively impact the gut microbiome." **(Page 5):**
Ruiz-Ojeda, F.J., Plaza-Díaz, J., Sáez-Lara, M.J., Gil, A. "Effects of Sweeteners on the Gut Microbiota: A Review of Experimental Studies and Clinical Trials." Advances in Nutrition. Pages S31–S48. First published January 2019, Retrieved from: https://doi.org/10.1093/advances/nmy037

"...150 to 700 times sweeter than regular sweeteners." **(Page 5):**
Strawbridge H. "Artificial sweeteners: sugar-free, but at what cost?" Harvard Health Publishing, Harvard Medical School. Last updated January 29, 2020. Retrieved from: https://www.health.harvard.edu/blog/artificial-sweeteners-sugar-free-but-at-what-cost-201207165030

ESSENTIAL INGREDIENTS

"...FDA requires an alcohol content of at least 35%." **(Page 14):**
Stanko, Caroline. "Does Vanilla Extract Contain Alcohol?" Taste of Home magazine. Published November 15, 2019. Retrieved from: https://www.tasteofhome.com/article/alcohol-in-extracts/

"Vanilla Extract." Food and Drug Administration. Code of Federal Regulations. Title 21, Volume 2. 21CFR169.175. Last revised April 1, 2019. Retrieved from: https://www.accessdata.fda.gov/scripts/cdrh/cfdocs/cfcfr/cfrsearch.cfm?fr=169.175

APPENDICES

APPENDIX 1

"…defined as five or more binge drinking episodes within the past month" (Page 161):
"Results from the 2018 National Survey on Drug Use and Health." Substance Abuse and Mental Health Services Administration (SAMHSA). Table 2.1B—Tobacco Product and Alcohol Use in Lifetime, Past Year, and Past Month among Persons Aged 12 or Older, by Age Group: Percentages, 2017 and 2018. Accessed December 2, 2019. Retrieved from: https://www.samhsa.gov/data/sites/default/files/cbhsq-reports/NSDUHDetailedTabs2018R2/NSDUHDetTabsSect2pe2018.htm#tab2-1b

"…this number rose by 58%" (Page 161):
Grant, B., Chou, S.P., Saha, T., et al. "Prevalence of 12-Month Alcohol Use, High-Risk Drinking, and DSM-IV Alcohol Use Disorder in the United States, 2001-2002 to 2012-2013: Results From the National Epidemiologic Survey on Alcohol and Related Conditions." JAMA Psychiatry. 74(9):911–923. Published September 6, 2017. Retrieved from: https://jamanetwork.com/journals/jamapsychiatry/fullarticle/2647079

"…appears to be on the rise both in the U.S. and globally." (Page 161):
"Results from the 2018 National Survey on Drug Use and Health." Substance Abuse and Mental Health Services Administration (SAMHSA). Table 2.1B—Tobacco Product and Alcohol Use in Lifetime, Past Year, and Past Month among Persons Aged 12 or Older, by Age Group: Percentages, 2017 and 2018. Accessed December 2, 2019. Retrieved from: https://www.samhsa.gov/data/sites/default/files/cbhsq-reports/NSDUHDetailedTabs2018R2/NSDUHDetTabsSect2pe2018.htm#tab2-1b

Manthey, J., Shield, K., Rylett, M., Hasan, O., Probst, C., Rehm, J. "Global alcohol exposure between 1990 and 2017 and forecasts until 2030: a modelling study." The Lancet. 393(10190): 2493-2503. Published May 07, 2019. Retrieved from: doi.org/10.1016/S0140-6736(18)32744-2

"…can be attributed to alcohol consumption." (Page 161):
"Alcohol and Public Health: Alcohol-Related Disease Impact (ARDI). Average for United States 2006–2010 Alcohol-Attributable Deaths Due to Excessive Alcohol Use." Centers for Disease Control and Prevention (CDC). Retrieved from: https://nccd.cdc.gov/DPH_ARDI/Default/Default.aspx

"…leading cause of death for people ages 15-49 years old." (Page 161):
GBD 2016 Global Collaborators. "Alcohol use and burden for 195 countries and territories, 1990–2016: a systematic analysis for the Global Burden of Disease Study 2016". The Lancet, volume 392, issue 10152, 1015-1035. Published August 23, 2018. Retrieved from: https://doi.org/10.1016/S0140-6736(18)31310-2

"…including heart disease, liver disease, and several types of cancer." (Page 161):
"Alcohol Use and Your Health." Centers for Disease Control and Prevention. Last reviewed December 30, 2019. Retrieved from: https://www.cdc.gov/alcohol/fact-sheets/alcohol-use.htm

"…when they were the same age." (Page 161):
Taylor, K. "Millennials are dragging down beer sales — but Gen Z marks a 'turning point' that will cause an even bigger problem for the industry." Business Insider. Published February 21, 2018. Retrieved from: https://www.businessinsider.com/millennials-gen-z-drag-down-beer-sales-2018-2

"...and diminished appeal." (Page 161):
Jones, D. "Gen Z - The Generation of Sobriety?" RDSI Research. Retrieved from: https://www.rdsiresearch.com/genz-the-generation-of-sobriety/

"...a spike in non-alcoholic beer sales." (Page 161):
Furnari, C. "Dry January Driving Sales of Non-Alcoholic Beers." Forbes. Published January 31, 2020. Retrieved from: https://www.forbes.com/sites/chrisfurnari/2020/01/31/dry-january-driving-increased-sales-of-non-alcoholic-beer/

"...develop zero-proof spirits." (Page 161):
Hartke, K. "Now, There is Zero-Proof that Alcohol Is What Makes a Great Cocktail." NPR. Published March 21, 2019. Retrieved from: https://www.npr.org/sections/thesalt/2019/03/21/701177978/now-there-is-zero-proof-that-alcohol-is-what-makes-a-great-cocktail

Açai (Page 162):
Zeratshy, K. "What are açai berries, and what are their health benefits?". Mayo Clinic. Published June 5, 2020. Retrieved from: http://www.mayoclinic.org/healthy-life-style/nutrition-and-healthy-eating/expert-answers/acai/faq-20057794

Sweeteners (Page 162):
Pope, E., Koren, G., Bozzo, P. "Sugar substitutes during pregnancy." Canadian Family Physician. 60(11):1003-1005. Published November 2014. Retrieved from: https://www.cfp.ca/content/60/11/1003

APPENDIX 2

Caffine (Page 162):
"Nutrition During Pregnancy. Frequently Asked Questions: Pregnancy." The American College of Obstetricians and Gynecologists. Copyright June 2020. Retrieved from: http://www.acog.org/patient-resources/faqs/pregnancy/nutrition-during-pregnancy

Herbal Teas (Page 162):
"Are Herbal Teas Safe During Your Pregnancy?". American Pregnancy Association. Retrieved from: https://americanpregnancy.org/pregnancy-health/herbal-tea/
https://www.nccih.nih.gov/health/lavender

ABOUT THE AUTHORS

Kerry Benson, MS, RD, LDN, is a registered dietitian and holds a master's degree in Nutritional Epidemiology from Tufts University. Prior to becoming a dietitian, she earned a master's degree in Behavioral Neuroscience and worked in a research lab for more than six years studying the effects of alcohol exposure during pregnancy on the developing brain. This experience sparked her interest in the topic of drinking, particularly in the context of pregnancy, and inspired her to embark on an alcohol-free journey. She is a licensed dietitian in the state of Pennsylvania and lives with her husband and two cats. She enjoys photography, staying active, cooking, and of course, trying out new alcohol-free products.

@healthycrayvings

Diana Licalzi, MS, RD, LDN, is a registered dietitian and holds a master's degree in Nutrition Science and Policy from Tufts University. Originally from Puerto Rico, Diana is dedicated to helping the Hispanic community meet its nutrition and health goals through her work in the diabetes community. She co-founded Reversing T2D, an online platform that helps individuals manage and reverse pre- and type 2 diabetes. Diana has also become very passionate about the "sober curious" movement. You can follow her on Instagram for alcohol-free advice, tips, and recipes.

@dietitian.diana